The 2027 Chiropractic Textbook

Volume 2

Claude Lessard, D.C.

© 2024

Dr. Claude Lessard

©2024 Claude Lessard, D.C.
www.LessardChiropractic.com
Lessard Chiropractic Center
210 Makefield Road, Morrisville, PA 19067
215-736-8816

The 2027 Chiropractic Textbook Volume 2

Dr. Claude Lessard

DEDICATION

IRENE GOLD, R.N., B.S., M.A., D.C.

I'll never think anything other than how, in 1973, a chance meeting at the corner of 72nd St. and Broadway in Manhattan held the seeds of change for my entire life.

I'd relocated from Québec to New York to begin studies in Pharmacology at St. John's University in Jamaica, NY. A few months into the curriculum, I realized this was not my path.

I encountered you as a vivacious ninth quarter student at Columbia Institute of Chiropractic.

On this day, having withdrawn from classes with what I thought to be a dream dissolving before my eyes, your enthusiasm in offering a glimpse into a different kind of dream was every bit life-giving.

And so it's been for more than 50 years: a long and storied career of Chiropractic seed – sowing. Yes, you had enthusiasm, but it was fueled by an unremitting desire to promote Chiropractic in a style eminently suited to the keen mind and immense generosity you possess.

Your joining the faculty at Sherman College enabled me to be one of a multitude of beneficiaries of your dedicated teaching skills. Not only did you help us through course curricula, but tirelessly over your professional career prepared us to pass the National Board of Chiropractic Examiners and bring Chiropractic to a waiting world.

I am honored to call you "friend". Your life has proven B.J.'s famous quote: "We never know how far reaching some thing we may think, say or do today, will affect the lives of millions tomorrow".

That word you spoke to me some 50 years ago is the same word you have spoken countless times to many, many others. Its ripple affects the lives and tomorrows of generations!

It is to you, Irene, that I dedicate Volume 2 of "The 2027 Chiropractic Textbook." Thank you for what you have chosen and continue to do with your life.

TABLE OF CONTENTS

DEDICATION TO IRENE GOLD, R.N., B.S., M.A., D.C.	V
PREFACE	1
CHIROPRACTIC LEXICON	3
GLOSSARY	3
INTRODUCTION TO VOLUME 2	10
ART. 103. CHIROPRACTIC CYCLES (DATA PROCESSING FLOWCHARTS)	10
ART. 104. HOW TO TELL THE NARRATIVE	11
ART. 105. PHYSIOLOGICAL CYCLES (FLOWCHARTS) IN THE BODY	11
ART. 106. NORMAL CYCLES (FLOWCHARTS)	12
ART. 107. ABNORMAL CYCLES (FLOWCHARTS)	12
ART. 108. COMPOUND OR COMPLEX CYCLES (FLOWCHARTS)	13
ART. 109. SPECIAL SENSE CYCLE (FLOWCHART)	15
ART. 110. THE CYCLE OF SIGHT	15
REVIEW QUESTIONS FOR ARTICLES 103 - 110	20
ART. 111. ABNORMAL SPECIAL SENSE CYCLE (FLOWCHART)	21
ART. 112. INTER-FIELD CYCLE (FLOWCHART)	21
ART. 113. THE UNIVERSAL DIAGRAM OF CYCLES (FLOWCHARTS)	23
ART. 114. A WRITTEN DIAGRAM SHOWING INNATE AND EDUCATED REALM	24
ART. 115. THE VERTEMERE CYCLE (FLOWCHART)	24
ART. 116. UNIVERSAL INFORMATION/F	25
ART. 117. INVASIVE INFORMATION/F	26
ART. 118. INNATE INFORMATION/F	26
ART. 119. INTERNAL RESISTANCE	26
ART. 120. TRAUMA	27
ART. 121. DISEASE AND DIS-EASE	27
REVIEW QUESTIONS FOR ARTICLES 111 - 121	29
ART. 122. THE CAUSE OF INCOORDINATION OF DIS-EASE	30
ART. 123. HOW THE CAUSE CAUSES INCOORDINATION *OF* DIS-EASE	30

ART. 124. THE ABNORMAL COMPLETE CYCLE CAUSING IN-COORDINATION OF ACTIVITIES 30

ART. 125. THE ABNORMAL SENSE CYCLE 31

ART. 127. OTHER USE OF THE NORMAL CYCLE FOR COORDINATION OF ACTIVITIES 34

ART. 128. HOW TO APPLY THE ABNORMAL CYCLE OF IN-COORDINATION OF ACTIVITIES 34

ART. 129. THE COMPLETE IN-COORDINATION OF ACTIVITIES CYCLE 35

ART. 130. "CONDITION" AND "LOCAL" 36

ART. 131. RESISTANCE 36

REVIEW QUESTIONS FOR ARTICLES 122 - 131 38

ART. 132. UNSOUNDNESS 39

ART. 133. SURVIVAL VALUES 39

ART. 134. ACCUMULATIVE CONSTRUCTIVE AND DECONSTRUCTIVE SURVIVAL VALUE 39

ART. 135. MOMENTUM 40

ART. 136. MOMENTUM AND TIMING REGARDING INCOORDINATION OF ACTIVITIES 40

ART. 137. MOMENTUM AND TIMING REGARDING COORDINATION OF ACTIVITIES 41

ART. 138. DEPLETION 42

ART. 139. DIMINUTION 42

ART. 140. REPLETION 42

ART. 141. DEGENERATION 42

REVIEW QUESTIONS FOR ARTICLES 132 - 141 44

ART. 142. THE CARRYING CAPABILITY OF NERVES 45

ART. 143. THE RESTORATION CYCLE FOR COORDINATION OF ACTIVITIES 48

ART. 144. THE PRACTICAL CYCLE FOR COORDINATION OF ACTIVIVITES 48

ART. 145. THE SEROUS CIRCULATION AS A MAJOR INSTRUMENT OF COORDINATION BY THE INNATE LAW 49

ART. 146. THE SEROUS CIRCULATION OF BODY CHEMISTRY 49

ART. 147. A CONTEMPORARY ANALOGY	52
ART. 148. CONDITION OF VITALITY	52
ART. 149. SEGMENTS OF THE SEROUS CIRCULATION OF BODY CHEMISTRY	52
ART. 150. THE EFFERENT SEROUS STREAM OF BODY CHEMISTRY	53
ART. 151. THE PERIPHERAL SEGMENT OF THE SEROUS CIRCULATION OF BODY CHEMISTRY	53
REVIEW QUESTIONS FOR ARTICLES 142 - 151	**56**
ART. 152. SERUM AND UREA	57
ART. 153. THE AFFERENT SEROUS STREAM	57
ART. 154. INNATE-LABORATORIES	57
ART. 155. THE POISON POSSIBILITIES OF SERUM	58
ART. 156. THE END OF THE SEROUS CYCLE	58
ART. 157. THE KIDNEYS	58
ART. 158. THE SKIN	59
ART. 159. EXCESS WATER SERUM (HYPERHYDRATION)	59
ART. 160. INSUFFICIENT WATER SERUM (DEHYDRATION)	59
ART. 161. EFFERENT SERUM POISONING	61
REVIEW QUESTIONS FOR ARTICLES 152 - 161	**62**
ART. 162. AFFERENT SERUM POISONING	63
ART. 163. UNSOUNDNESS FROM EXCESS WATER SERUM	63
ART. 164. UNSOUNDNESS FROM INSUFFICIENT WATER SERUM	63
ART. 165. A CHIROPRACTIC DISCOVERY	63
WORLD AND LIFE VIEW POINTS	**64**
ART. 166. POISON	67
ART. 167. THE POSSIBILITIES OF POISON	67
ART. 168. WHAT WE KNOW ABOUT POISONS	67
ART. 169. WHAT WE DO NOT KNOW ABOUT POISONS	68
ART. 170. HOW OUR COLLECTIVE EDUCATED INTELLIGENCE FOUND OUT ABOUT POISON SUBSTANCES	68
ART. 171. SENTIENT COMPUTATION OF BIOLOGICAL PROCESSES OF POISON	69
REVIEW QUESTIONS FOR ARTICLES 162 - 171	**70**

ART. 172. SOME ACCUMULATED KNOWLEDGE OF POISONS	71
ART. 173. FOOD	71
ART. 174. DIET	72
ART. 175. GOOD EDUCATED CHOICE OF NUTRITION BASED ON NATURAL HUNGER, NATURAL CRAVINGS, NATURAL THIRST, AND NATURAL DESIRES IS ADIO	73
ART. 176. THE PARADOX OF THE COLLECTIVE EDUCATED CONTROL OF ALWAYS CHOOSING ABOVE-DOWN-INSIDE-OUT VERSUS SOMETIMES CHOOSING OUTSIDE-IN-BELOW-UP	74
ART. 177. EXERCISE	76
ART. 178. HYGIENE	76
ART. 179. THE POISONS OF ENVIRONMENT	77
ART. 180. WATER, AIR, SUNLIGHT, AND CLIMATE AS ENVIRONMENT FACTORS	77
ART. 181. FOOD AS AN ENVIRONMENTAL FACTOR	79
REVIEW QUESTIONS FOR ARTICLES 172 - 181	80
ART. 182. AIR AS ENVIRONMENTAL FACTOR	81
ART. 183. CLIMATE AS A FACTOR OF ENVIRONMENT	81
ART. 184. HYGIENE AND SANITATION AS ENVIRONMENTAL FACTORS	81
ART. 185. EFFLUVIA AS AN ENVIRONMENTAL FACTOR	82
ART. 186. GERMS AS A FACTOR OF ENVIRONMENT	82
ART. 187. PARASITES	83
ART. 188. EPIDEMICS, ENDEMICS, AND PANDEMICS	84
ART. 189. CONTAGION AND INFECTION	84
ART. 190. BLOOD POISON	84
ART. 191. IMMUNITY	84
REVIEW QUESTIONS FOR ARTICLES 182 - 191	86
ART. 192. DIS-EASE AND ITS CAUSE IS CONTINUALLY IN A STATE OF FLUX	87
ART. 193. THE PHILOSOPHY OF ADAPTIVE BODY CHEMISTRY	88
ART. 194. ADAPTIVE BODY CHEMISTRY CYCLE AND PROCESSING OF TOXINS	88
ART. 195. IMBALANCE OF BODY CHEMISTRY	88
ART. 196. UN-ADAPTED BODY ACTIVITIES	89

ART. 197. STIMULATION 89

ART. 198. INHIBITION 89

ART. 199. APPLICATION OF THE CYCLES OF THE BODY'S ADAPTABILITY TO POISON 89

ART. 200. APPLICATION OF CYCLES OF THE BODY'S UNADAPTABILITY TO POISON DUE TO LIMITATION OF E/MATTER 91

ART. 201. POISON IS ALWAYS AN EXTERNAL INVASIVE INFORMATION/F 93

REVIEW QUESTIONS FOR ARTICLES 192 - 201 94

ART. 202. ADDICTION AND HABIT 95

ART. 204. MEDICATION HABITS AND PAIN KILLERS ADDICTION 96

ART. 205. 100%/PERFECT INSTANTANEOUS INTEGRAL ADAPTATION 96

ART. 206. ADAPTATION 97

ART. 207. GENETIC SUSCEPTIBILITY 98

REVIEW QUESTIONS FOR ARTICLES 202 - 207 99

BIBLIOGRAPHY VOL 2: 100

CURRICULUM VITAE
DR. CLAUDE LESSARD 101

Dr. Claude Lessard

PREFACE

This is a series of four academic volumes to be studied as part of the chiropractic curriculum for the student to learn chiropractic and graduate as a chiropractor. It is the 2027 reconstructed version of its original precursor, *"CHIROPRACTIC TEXT BOOK"* written by Ralph W. Stephenson, D.C. in 1927. This is the second volume of the series, what Stephenson calls the "Sophomore Text." Portions of this volume are taken directly from the original text and updated with NEW knowledge produced from NEW information of the last hundred years. The same building blocks of chiropractic are refashioned into a contemporary context that includes 130 years of continuous discoveries. Credit is given to D.D. Palmer, D.C., B.J. Palmer, D.C. and R.W. Stephenson, D.C. We all stand on their shoulders as we move forward.

I applied to Sherman College in December of 1973. I was first introduced to the founder of Sherman College, Thom Gelardi, D.C. during the orientation day. Over the years, Thom and I developed a close relationship. After hundreds of hours of conversation, it was at his suggestion, in the early summer of 2021 that I undertook the task of rewriting the chiropractic textbook.

I owe much to Reggie Gold, D.C. for facilitating the formation of my chiropractic mind and for always encouraging me to THINK and THINK and THINK. I am grateful to Reggie for his constant challenges that stretched me to this day to grasp the unadulterated aspect of the exclusivity of the chiropractic objective.

I have no doubt that without the constant affirmation, encouragement, and deep friendship of Joseph Strauss, D.C., *The 2027 Chiropractic Textbook* could never have been rewritten.

My heartfelt gratitude goes James Healey, D.C. for continuously being my devil's advocate, asking the questions that provide a needed accuracy check to my philosophical contemplation. His constant desire for accurate articulation to facilitate understanding is a true inspiration. Thank you, Jim.

Thank you to Tom Gregory, D.C. for your steady listening and comments on the philosophical accuracy of the text.

Thank you Jack Bourla, D.C. for the specific chiropractic editing of Volume 2 into a comprehensive academic text. Your questions have helped me clarify some of the more difficult concepts to understand. Your contributions have greatly enriched the text.

Thank you Judy Campanale, D.C. for providing me with my weekly spinal checks. I am eternally grateful to you for so many long hours of meaningful conversation about new insights that were instrumental in writing Volume 2.

I owe my grateful thanks to Amanda Janiec for overseeing the entire project and making it possible. As Amanda tackled the English editing of the manuscripts with judicious research for the proper references in the texts, making sure I was accurate, she became my radar following the text through her scholarly perspective. Thank you Amanda, for your dedication and for sharing your educated expertise.

Finally, to the one and only person who saw me through it all, Sara, my spouse of fifty years without whom I could not be the person that I am today. From the very beginning of translating my phonetic notes of our first quarter at Sherman, she never wavered and has always been true. I love you, Sara.

These volumes are mainly *"The Chiropractic Text Book"* originally written by R.W. Shephenson, D.C. They include error corrections and are updated with NEW knowledge of the past hundred years.

Dr. Claude Lessard

The instructions contained therein are further developed from the original concepts of the founder of chiropractic, Daniel David Palmer, D.C. and his son, the developer of chiropractic, Bartlett Joshua Palmer, D.C. Within these volumes, the falsification and deconstruction of the theistic and anthropomorphic characters given to some of the chiropractic's scientific principles and scientific laws, namely universal intelligence and innate intelligence, are proven. Those chiropractic concepts are then reconstructed on the solid bedrock of the testable and verifiable principles of chiropractic's basic science; they include new information acquired since 1927 that dictates the chiropractic objective. These four volumes contain NEW knowledge that has been discovered and constructed, within the past 100 years, from NEW information that was unavailable from 1895 to 1927 and beyond. They cover the philosophy, the science, and the art of chiropractic. They are intended to be a further study of chiropractic that is continuously developed to **CARRY ON** the genius of our predecessors, D.D. and B.J. Palmer into the twenty first century; they are designed to convey more precisely "WHAT" chiropractic is, "HOW" to apply its scientific principles, and the **hard to vary explanation** of "WHY" chiropractic is an evolutionary humanitarian approach to EVERY experience of life, not just the experience of health. These volumes comprise error corrections that are necessary for the student to obtain an assured confidence in the chiropractic objective including its universal value. They honor yet modernize this significant discovery and the greater understanding of its necessary and humanitarian service to the world. It was Joseph B. Strauss, D.C. who wrote in 2002, "I do not believe that you can truly understand chiropractic philosophy without studying Stephenson. There are truths within and errors that need to be seen and understood for any student to ever begin to reach a level of comprehension of chiropractic as it was and is today."[1] Students are encouraged to study Stephenson's textbook of 1927, ALL of the Strauss' Blue Books, and the two Blue Books that I have personally authored, *A New Look at Chiropractic's Basic Science* and *Timed Out: Chiropractic*.

It is the hope that the truths and error corrections contained within the pages of these volumes will inform and inspire future generations of chiropractors so that they can make an informed choice in constructing their professional mission. Based on the study of the 33 principles of chiropractic's basic science, it is clear that the sole aim of the chiropractic objective is, EXCLUSIVELY, the restoration of normal transmission of innate impulses through the location, analysis, and the facilitation of the correction of vertebral subluxations. PERIOD.

These texts have been written for educational instruction. They are divided into Volume One (First Year Chiropractic Text), Volume Two (Second Year Chiropractic Text), Volume Three (Third Year Chiropractic Text), and Volume Four (Fourth Year Chiropractic Text). Following the original layout of Stephenson's Text Book allows for the integral comparison of topics. There are questions for review that are intended to help the student THINK and "internalize" the value of chiropractic, and raise inquiry to test any of its 33 scientific principles in order to verify or falsify any of them. The student is urged to become familiar with the unique chiropractic lexicon at the beginning of every volume in order to properly understand the meaning of those terms that will undoubtedly assist the study of the text. Hopefully, these four volumes of the updated chiropractic textbook will encourage future chiropractors to CARRY ON and further develop chiropractic, that will include NEW knowledge, insights, and error corrections into the third millennium and forever more.

---

1. Strauss, Joseph. "The Green Book Commentaries, Vol. XIV (1927) Chiropractic Text Book.: Levittown, PA: Foundation for Advancement of Chiropractic Education. (2002) p. 17

CHIROPRACTIC LEXICON

GLOSSARY

In order to continue to explore the previously established central core of chiropractic, namely its principles and tenets, in a contemporary way we must rely on a base set terminology. As we move forward our educated intelligence grows and it requires that we progress without condemnation. The following glossary of terms was compiled, with the help of Joe Strauss, D.C., many of which are originally from Stephenson's text. Some additional terms that are uniquely needed for practicing the chiropractic objective have been incorporated.

100%/perfect: A quality of being free from all flaws or defect. It is the fullness of something material or immaterial.

Adaptability (sign of life): The intrinsic ability that a living organism possesses to act on all information/force, which comes to it whether innate or universal.

Adaptation: The movement of a living organism or any of its parts, or the structural change in that organism, to use or to circumvent environmental information/force. Adaptation is a continuous process — continually varying, it is never constant and unvarying, as are other universal laws. Adaptation is a universal principle — the only one of its kind. It is the principle of change and the change is always according to law, which is 100%/perfect instantaneous integral adaptation.

ADIO (Acronym for Above-Down-Inside-Out):

    1. An exclusive model of world viewpoint, under which chiropractic philosophy, logically and uncompromisingly, exists.

    2. A thinking process with a unique perspective on life. First, there are absolutes in life (Prin. 1, 6, 20). Second, everything has a cause that should be addressed, if possible (Prin. 17, 24). Third, there is a pre-eminence to the educated intelligence of humankind (Prin. 22, 27), a 100%/perfect universal intelligence (Prin. 1,5).

    3. Life comes from universal organization ABOVE (Prin. 1, 3), DOWN to living things' innate adaptation (Prin. 20, 23), expressing signs of life INSIDE the body (Prin. 18), to be manifested OUT as a living entity (Prin. 21).

    4. In regards to coordination of activities of body parts (Prin. 32), in the vertebrate body, the innate impulse flows from the brain cell ABOVE (Prin. 28), DOWN to the tissue cell below (Prin. 18), is expressed from INSIDE the body part (Prin. 21), to be manifested OUT as coordinative purpose (Prin. 21, 32), according to universal laws (Prin. 24).

ADIO analysis: A specific method of chiropractic analysis based on the principles i.e., that the function of the innate law is always normal (Prin. 27); that the innate law will adapt and organize para-vertebral muscles to process a vertebral adjustment, thus correcting a vertebral subluxation to restore to innate-normal the transmission of innate impulses for coordination of activities within the limitation of E/matter (Prin. 23, 24, 31a, 31b). The chiropractor's pre-check is to palpate and identify the vectors of the correcting muscles of a vertebral subluxation used by the innate law, which reveal when and where a vertebral subluxation exists, for the appropriate introduction of a specific adjustic thrust to facilitate the processing of a vertebral adjustment by the innate law. The chiropractor's post-check is to palpate those same muscles to determine if the vertebral subluxation has been corrected.

Adjustic thrust: An adjustic thrust is a specific, external, educated information/force introduced at the site of a subluxated vertebra with the intent to be adapted by the innate law of living things to perform a vertebral adjustment.

Afferent nerve: The nerve that transmit trophic impulses from receptor tissue cell to central processing brain cell for coordination of activities. It is the route of feedback information/force from tissue cell to brain cell. It not to be confused with sensory nerves, which transmit sensory impulses from sense organs to physical brain.

Analytical post-check: The end-point of a chiropractic analysis to determine if the correction of a vertebral subluxation has occurred. It is the COMPLETION of practicing the chiropractic objective.

Analytical pre-check: The start-point of a chiropractic analysis that locates and identify the correcting muscles of a vertebral subluxation in order to introduce to it a specific adjustic thrust to facilitate its correction by the innate law.

Assimilation (sign of life): The ability of a living organism to selectively take food materials into its body and make them a part of itself according to a systematic program designed by a universal intelligence.

Characterization: The construction of specific codes by the universal principle of organization that organizes universal information/force in order to maintain energy/matter in existence; it is also the reconstruction (modified for living energy/matter) of specific codes by the innate law of living things that adapts universal information/force into innate information/force.

Chiropractic analysis: A chiropractic analysis is the act of surveying the vertebral column in detail, to locate and identify the vectors of the corrective muscles working to correct a vertebral subluxation, in order to introduce a specific adjustic thrust to facilitate the processing of a vertebral adjustment by the innate law.

Chiropractic Meaning of Existence: It is the expression of the universal principle of organization through ALL energy/matter, living and non-living.

Chiropractic objective: The chiropractic objective is to locate, analyze, and facilitate the correction of vertebral subluxations for an innate-normal transmission of the innate impulses of the body. PERIOD. The chiropractic objective is derived directly from the thirty-three principles of chiropractic's basic science. Nothing more. Nothing less. Nothing else.

Chiropractor: One who knows the science, art and philosophy of Chiropractic and how to adjust subluxated vertebrae by placing in apposition the articular processes of the vertebral column.[2]

Chiropractor's vision: The chiropractor's vision is to insure the availability of chiropractic care to EVERYONE now and forever.

Coding: The assignment of specific characters to identify a specific communication system programmed to construct a message.

---

2. Palmer, B.J., "The Science of Chiropractic, Its Principles and Philosophies." 4th Ed., Davenport, IA: The Palmer School of Chiropractic - Chiropractic Fountain Head. (1920) p. 12

Computation: The operation of a computing system. It is the processing of data of a computing system using a software program (Prin. 5).

Copyability: The ability to be copied, to be duplicatable. From the maxim that "One cannot give what one does not have." Every human invention is a copy of something already existing in principle. The universe is complete.

Counterfactuals: They are facts not about what is "actual" but about what is possible or not possible. For example, Dead Sea scrolls exist somewhere "hidden" on our planet. That is a physical property of those scrolls since they do exist. That it ***could be possible*** to read the words on them is a counterfactual property regardless of whether those scrolls would ever be discovered. And yet that those words ***could be*** read would still be true.

De-coding: To convert a coded message into intelligible language that can be understood.

Disease and DIS-EASE: Disease is a term used by physicians for sickness. To them it is an entity and is worthy of a name, hence diagnosis. DIS-EASE is a chiropractic term meaning not having ease; or lack of ease. It is lack of an entity. It is a condition of energy/matter when it does not have the property of ease. Ease is the entity, and DIS-EASE the lack of it.

E/matter: This term means energy-matter. Since $E=mc^2$, energy and matter are interchangeable; energy is simply a different configuration (properties) of electrons, protons, and neutrons with varying velocities (activities). For example, water has 2 molecules of hydrogen and 1 molecule of oxygen, whether it is in a fluid state, solid state, or vapor state. It is dependent upon the movement of its basic elements. It is a term reminding us that energy and matter are interchangeable as per $E=mc^2$, and that matter is comprised of electrons, protons, and neutrons configured at less than the square of the speed of light.

Educated brain/field: That part of the body used by innate law of living things, as an organ, for reason, will, memory, education, and the voluntary functions.

Educated control: Educated control (also known as educated mind) is the activity of innate law of living things in the educated brain/field as an organ. The output of this activity is educated impulses such as thoughts, reasoning, will, memory, etc.… The innate law of living things controls the functions of the voluntary systems via the educated brain. Educated impulses are modified innate impulses that have passed through the educated brain and are mostly for adaptation to things external to the body.

Educated impulse: The innate information/force through the educated brain/field that becomes modified with whatever quality the educated mind/control can give it for the voluntary functions of the body. Note that the educated brain "controls" nothing, except that the innate information/force passes through it. Adaptation of information/force is ALWAYS and ONLY through the coding of innate impulses by the innate law. When innate impulses pass through the educated brain, they are "tinctured" and modified into educated impulses so there can be conscious action.

Educated Intelligence: The capability of the educated brain/field to function. It starts at 0% at birth and reaches its maximum limit at the death of the body (since it will develop no further).

Educated information/force: Educated information/force is innate information/force that has been modified by the educated control for voluntary functions. It is really an educated impulse.

Efferent nerve: The transmitting nerve of innate impulses from the central processing brain cell to the receptor tissue cell. It is the route of conducted innate information/force from brain cell to tissue cell.

Dr. Claude Lessard

Energy: Electrons, protons, and neutrons configured at the square of the speed of light ($E=mc^2$).

E/matter: Energy/matter is electrons, protons, and neutrons configured at specific velocities in time.

Existence: The continuous motion of elemental particles of E/matter.

External educated information/force: An external educated information/force is innate information/force that has been voluntarily modified by the educated intelligence with a new educated character for so called voluntary action with a definite purpose. Ex: An adjustic thrust.

Flow: The action of something moving along in a steady continuous stream. In the body, it is the smooth continuous movement of conducted information/F from one place to another.

Growth (sign of life): Growth is the ability of a living organism to expand according to intelligent programming to mature in size and is dependent upon the power of assimilation.

Hard to vary explanation: An explanation that provides specific details that fit together so tightly that it is impossible to change any detail without affecting its whole. In the case of chiropractic, the principles of its basic science are the hard to vary explanation of chiropractic.

Impression: It is the information/force coded by the innate law as trophic impulses, based on the complexity of the tissue cell concerning its soundness and functions.

Information/F: Information/force are computed and coded instructions to configure electrons, protons, neutrons, and their velocities.

Inforuns: Inforuns, (also known as foruns) are non-discrete information/force units that are continually organized by the universal principle of organization providing properties and actions to all E/matter in order to *maintain* it in existence (Prin. 1, 8). Inforuns must be adapted by the innate law of living things and constructed into innate impulses for coordination of activities of all the parts of the body, or into innate rays/waves for cellular metabolism in order to *maintain* E/matter alive (Prin. 21, 23).

Innate control: Innate control (also known as innate mind) is the activity of the innate law in the innate field. It is the introduction of innate instructive information/F, as governance, into E/matter via the innate field of the body of **living** things to **maintain** the material of the body alive within the limits of adaptation (Prin. 21, 24).

Innate field: The innate field (also know as innate brain) is:
   a) That aspect of the living body used by the innate law of living things, as an operating system, in which to adapt universal information/F and assemble them,

   b) That facet of a living organism controlled by the innate law of living things, as an operating system, in which to assemble innate impulses, innate rays or innate waves, trophic impulses, and sensory impulses.

Innate impulse: Innate impulse (also known as mental impulse) is unit of information/F for a specific body part, for a specific function, for coordination of activities. A specific instruction given to a body part, for coordination of activities, for the present moment.

Innate information/F: Innate information/force (also known as innate force) is universal information/force adapted by the innate law of living things and codified for use in the body. It is assembled for dynamic functional process to cause tissue cells to function or to offer resistance to the environment. It is transmitted by nerve conduction from the brain to the tissue cell and is called an ***innate impulse*** when it impels parts of the body for coordinated action; it is called an ***educated impulse*** for voluntary actions; it is called a ***trophic impulse*** for feedback from the state and functions of body parts to the brain; when it is radiated from within all cells of the body for metabolism it is called an ***innate ray/wave***; and it is called a ***sensory impulse*** when it is transmitted by sensory nerve from sense organs to the brain for adaptation to the environment. It is constructive toward structural E/matter (Prin. 26). Chiropractic ONLY addresses the innate impulse. Chiropractic does NOT address the educated impulse, the trophic impulse, the innate ray/wave or the sensory impulse.

Innate law of living things: The innate law of living (also known as innate intelligence) is the inborn organizing principle governing the body of a living thing through adaptation in order to **maintain** it alive, only if it is possible according to universal laws. It is the essential extension of the universal principle of organization that is expressed through living E/matter keeping it alive through multiple levels of complex organization. It implements design, programming, self-correction, adjustability and adaptation to internal and external effectors.

Innate ray/wave: A unit of information/F for a specific tissue cell unit to keep it metabolically sound and alive for a specific unit of time within limitations of E/matter.

Instantaneous integral adaptation: Instantaneous integral adaptation (also known as intellectual adaptation) is the 100%/perfect cooperative processes of the innate law of living things to compute ways and means of adapting universal information/F and E/matter for use in the body and for coordination of activities. The interoperability of the innate law, in the innate field, to keep ALL the complexities of the living things organized to **maintain** it alive if it is possible according to universal laws (Prin. 21, 23, 24).

Instantiation: The act of producing a specific application of a principle. It is a process to deduce an individual statement from a general principle; the representation of an idea in the form of an instance of it.

Interoperability: A characteristic of the innate law in the innate field adapting information/F, the interface of which is completely understood to work with ALL the systems of the body, at present or in the future, moment to moment in either implementation or access.

Intra-cell particulates: Components of a cell adapted through innate information/F, in the form of innate rays/waves, that have been specifically coded by the innate law to process innate-normal metabolism (Prin. 27) for soundness of the cell.

Invasive information/F: Universal information/F acting powerfully upon tissue in spite of the innate resistance of the body, or in cases where the resistance of the body is lowered.

Matter: Electrons, protons, and neutrons configured at *less* that the square of the speed of light.

Mission of the chiropractic profession: The mission of the chiropractic profession is the specific task of increasing the awareness of the UNIVERSAL values of chiropractic for EVERYONE through education and by practicing the chiropractic objective.

Modifier: A slight change transforming a specific code through educated control that tincture innate impulses into educated impulses for voluntary functions.

Momentum: The possession of motion that is compounded by the mass of E/matter moved and its velocity. It is the active movement of E/matter in time. In chiropractic, momentum is the active frequencies of motion of the transmitting E/matter (neuron-transmitters) within the vertebrate body. Mass x Velocity = Momentum. Also momentum is subject to interference through being transferred from one element of information/F to another by vertebral subluxations. The *total* momentum of E/matter of the living body is always conserved.

Motor nerve: The nerve that transmits educated impulses (modified innate impulses) from the central processing brain cell to the receptor tissue cell. It is the route of educated functions from brain cell to tissue cell for voluntary actions.

Myo-vector: A chiropractic term describing the directional work of an operating para-vertebral muscle, adapted by the innate law, to process a vertebral adjustment for the correction of a vertebral subluxation within the limitations of E/matter (Prin. 23, 24, 31a, 31b). Utilized in ADIO analysis, a myo-vector reveals that the vertebra is not, at that moment, correctly positioned and is interfering with the transmission of innate impulses.

Objective chiropractor (OC): An Objective Chiropractor is one WHO chooses to practice EXCLUSIVELY the chiropractic objective and nothing else.

Penetrative information/F: Invasive information/F that acts powerfully assailing the body and that has effect upon tissue in spite of the innate resistance of the body.

Physical brain: That part of the central nerve system used by the innate law of living things, as an organ, to centralize innate impulses that will be conducted across nerves for distribution to all the parts of the body for coordination of actions. It is also the organ of adaptation including the faculties of memory, will, and reason.

Poison: Any substance introduced into or manufactured within the living body, which the innate law of living things cannot process for metabolism.

Principle: A fundamental truth that is the foundation of universal laws.

Purpose of chiropractic: The purpose of chiropractic is to restore the momentum of transmission of innate impulses through the location, analysis and facilitation of the correction of vertebral subluxations.

Resistive information/F: Internal innate information/F that opposes invasive or penetrative information/F. It may manifests in many forms, physical, chemical, or mechanical. It is not called resistive information/F unless it is of that character. It is necessary for keeping ALL information/F in balance within the body.

Sensory nerve: The nerve that transmits sensory impulses from the perceptible tissue cell sensor to the brain cell processor. It is the route of special sense functions from the external impressions detected by a tissue cell sensor to a brain cell processor to adapt to the environment. Not to be confused with the afferent nerves used for feedback for coordination of activities.

Tone: "Tone is the normal degree of **nerve** tension. Tone is expressed in functions by the normal elasticity, activity, strength and excitability [of **nerves** which are] too tense or too slack".[25] Tone is the degree of ease manifested by the neurons that are engaged in the transmission of innate impulses.

Trophic impulse/signal: Information/F that has been characterized and coded by the innate law providing specific feedback information of the metabolic and coordinative state of a tissue cell. A trophic impulse/signal is transmitted through afferent nerves from tissue cell to brain cell via its cell body waving

---

25. Palmer. D.D., "Text-Book of the Science, Art, and Philosophy of Chiropractic for Students and Practioners." Portland, OR: Portland Printing House Company. (1910) p.7

it signal through the innate field for coordination of activities. Not to be confused with the sensory nerves.

Universal information/F: Information/F organized **by** the universal principle of organization that is manifested by physical laws; it provides properties and actions to all E/matter that maintains it in existence; it is deconstructive toward structural E/matter (Prin. 26).

Universal intelligence: The fundamental CAUSE in chiropractic. Philosophically, it is the capability of the universal principle of organization to organize all of the infinite information/F, in the universal field to provide the properties and the actions of all E/matter **maintaining** it in existence (Prin. 1). It is the cause of organization due to the fact that organization bespeaks intelligence.

Universal principle of organization: The fundamental principle (major premise) of chiropractic's basic science intrinsic to all E/matter. The universal principle of organization is continually organizing all E/matter supplying properties and actions to all E/matter in order to maintain it in existence. It is the initial condition of chiropractic's basic science that organizes E/matter maintaining it in existence.

Vertebral adjustment and chiropractic adjustment: A vertebral adjustment is the correction of a vertebral subluxation caused by the process of adapting information/F by the innate law of living things. A chiropractic adjustment is the application of an adjustic thrust by a chiropractor, at the specific site of a vertebral subluxation, with the intent that the innate law will adapt this specific educated information/F to process a vertebral adjustment.

Vertebral subluxation: A vertebral subluxation is the condition of a vertebra that has lost its proper juxtaposition with the one above or the one below, or both; to an extent less than a luxation; which impinges nerves and interferes with the transmission of innate impulses.

Viability: The capability of E/matter to live.

Vibration: The motion of a tissue cell performing its function.

Vitality: The soundness or integrity of a tissue cell. It is the quality of liveliness of a cell.

Dr. Claude Lessard

INTRODUCTION TO VOLUME 2

As explained in Volume 1, the universe is continually maintained in existence through the universal principle of organization. It is the initial condition and it is the fundamental principle of chiropractic's basic science (Prin. 1). Through rational logic and deductive reasoning this major premise cascades into 32 subsequent principles forming a solid platform into a bedrock on which chiropractic is constructed. From divided to condensed, from living and thinking E/matter, the rational trajectory is progressing to an increase in complexity through this universal principle of organization and its essential extended continuation, called the innate law of living things.

Volume 2 is the study of cycles (universal and bio-data processing flowcharts) from the state of E/matter for the purpose of a greater understanding of the intrinsic working knowledge of the organizing principle. The study of cycles is the arbitrary operation of steps and/or processes involved concerning the multiple levels of organization of E/matter based on the principles of chiropractic's basic science. We will look deeply at different cycles from a chiropractic philosophy perspective; we will study normal cycle, abnormal cycle, vertemere cycle, vertebral subluxation cycle, restoration cycle, inter-field cycle, etc. This chiropractic perspective is vitalistic and is an altogether different perspective than the mechanists. Chiropractic has a responsibility to teach its curriculum from a vitalistic viewpoint. It should enable active learning that trains the mind to think, via a faculty that will facilitate a chiropractic integration of the material presented, not only instill the information. Unless this occurs, it will be a copy of the medical mechanistic model which is based on treating effects. Chiropractic is always about correcting a cause, not effects. Chiropractic institutions must be free to direct, without outside interference, those functions that may from time to time, challenge, but ultimately will enrich chiropractic.

We will spend a considerable amount of time on the subject of cycles, because for E/matter to live, it needs first to be maintained in existence. It is just one of several prerequisites. However, it is far from sufficient to even begin to appreciate the innate law of living things. You need to be thoroughly familiar with cycles and how they relate to the principles of chiropractic's basic science. Since chiropractic is a "work in progress", this breathtaking panorama provides a vision, looking toward the horizon of a humanitarian approach to experience life through the practice of the chiropractic objective. The articles continue to be numbered from where Volume 1 left off and employs the same method.

ART. 103. CHIROPRACTIC CYCLES (DATA PROCESSING FLOWCHARTS)

In chiropractic, cycles are the explanation of the successive steps that are infinitely continual, without beginning and/or end, according to universal laws. The starting point of cycles begins from cause to effects and back again to cause within a specific field of endeavor. They are agents of the innate law of living things to compute processes for coherence within the body (Prin. 33). As far as living E/matter is concerned, cycles start at the moment the living body has begun construction, and end with its deconstruction. Its return to universal elements of E/matter signals a continual maintaining of E/matter's existence (Prin. 1). For this reason, cycles are operating from the multilevel states of organization of E/matter as it is continually maintained in existence. Volume 2 teaches a broader idea of cycles than was provided in Volume 1. In the work of Volume 1, the simple cycle and the normal complete cycle for coordination of activities were given, and their narratives pertained to what happens when the innate law controls and governs the human body. Whereas, chiropractic cycles encompass a much broader field. They pertain to the narratives of the cause of continuity about anything, anywhere, in the universe, from the chiropractic standpoint of reasoning, such as, the fundamental organizing principle maintaining all of the universe in existence, the innate law of living things maintaining

E/matter alive for a lifetime if it is possible within the limitations of E/matter. In particular, those cycles pertain to the processes resulting in the coherence that fulfills the principle of coordination of action (Prin. 32), and to a specific cause of interference in transmission of conducted information/F (Prin. 29, 30, 31a) that unites the non-material with the material, the non-discrete with the discrete (Prin. 10). Within the body of living vertebrates, this interference is caused by the vertebral subluxation, which in sequence violates the principle of coordination.

ART. 104. HOW TO TELL THE NARRATIVE

The narrative is the "hard to vary" explanation based on the principles of chiropractic's basic science of the cyclic processes, and it may be reversed, going from the effect to the cause and from cause back to effect. This feature of the narrative can happen only for coordination of activities of all the body parts. One must realize that once the universal principle of organization (Prin. 1) was designed and programmed by a universal intelligence, it continues perfectly and infinitely. For this reason, when we speak of cause and effect, it is arbitrary and it is contained within the unlimited continuity of an infinite cycle.

Philosophically, we always start reasoning somewhere that is consistent with rational logic. Therefore, chiropractic's basic science starts with an initial principle of universal organization (Prin. 1) that has been designed and programmed by a universal intelligence. According to chiropractic philosophy, this universal principle of organization is an effect of a universal intelligence. For chiropractic, this means that whenever we work with cycles, we assume an "a priori" statement and we assign it a causality that initiates the beginning of chiropractic cycles. Every field of endeavor must assume a theory, in order to start somewhere that will eventually be tested to verify and demonstrate its veracity or falsification.

In the normal complete cycle for coordination of activities of the body parts, the cause is the innate law of living things (Prin. 20), which is an essential continuous extension of the universal principle of organization (Prin. 1). In the normal special sense cycles, the cause is the universal principle of organization (Prin. 1) maintaining the environment in existence and the innate law (Prin. 20) maintaining some of the environment alive within the limits of adaptation (Prin. 24). In the abnormal cycle responsible for in-coordination of activities, the cause is the vertebral subluxation (Prin. 30, 31a). In the restoration cycle for coordination of activities, the cause of this restoration is the correction of the vertebral subluxation by the innate law (Prin. 31b). In chiropractic, philosophically speaking, a universal intelligence is the cause of the universal principle of organization and is also the ultimate cause of all cycles. I must point out that this universal intelligence has also a cause and that this cause is outside the realm of chiropractic philosophy. It is in the realm of theology. Chiropractic is not theology. Chiropractic is philosophy, science, and art *(See Art. 2).*

ART. 105. PHYSIOLOGICAL CYCLES (FLOWCHARTS) IN THE BODY

The serous cycle is the circulation of the fluids of the body. It is mainly the afferent cycle of the circulation of body chemistry for elimination of waste materials.

The blood cycle is the circulation of blood in a cyclic course. It is mainly the efferent cycle of body chemistry for metabolic nutrition.

The respiration cycle is the course of air into an out of the lungs, and the course of the oxygen to the periphery and back again to the environment.

The nutrition cycle is the course of food from the environment to the digestive track, then to the periphery and back to the environment again.

The caloric cycle is the generation, distribution, and dissipation of heat.

The nerve cycle is the arrangement of nerve tissue from brain to periphery and back again to brain including trophic impulse/signal waves for coordination of activities of body parts, educated impulses for voluntary actions and sensory impulses for sensory input.

The study of these cycles is found in and forms the basis for chiropractic physiology from a vitalistic perspective. In particular, the innate law is a fundamental and vital principle, which is an essential continuous extension of the universal principle of organization (designed and programmed by a universal intelligence). The innate law maintains E/matter alive for its lifetime through the adaptation of information/F and E/matter for use in the body, so that all body parts have coordination of action for mutual benefit within limitations of E/matter (Prin. 20, 21, 23, 24).

ART. 106. NORMAL CYCLES (FLOWCHARTS)

Normal cycles are those in which the orderly and normal sequencing processes are unbroken, signifying that all processes are in perfect coherence and in perfect harmony. The cause in normal cycles is in the interface between the non-discrete and the discrete. It is information/F that unites the non-material with the material (Prin. 10) that generates the cycles of motion (Prin. 15). The simple cycle and the normal complete cycle for coordination of activities are the most studied cycles in chiropractic. Normal cycles are the study of normality, which is truly innate-normal (Prin. 27). The question of abnormality does not enter, except for comparison. It is for this reason that the chiropractic objective is exclusively about the location, analysis, and facilitation of the correction of vertebral subluxations for the restoration in transmission of innate impulses.

All the work in Volume 1, regarding cycles, was the study of normality. When abnormality was mentioned or described, it was in comparison or for further explanation of the normal. According to the Merriam-Webster dictionary, normal means, running true to form, not exhibiting defect or irregularity. It is necessary for us to understand normality before we can understand abnormality. The normal sequencing processes of cycles, in chiropractic, are a vitalistic explanation of human physiology. From a chiropractic standpoint it demonstrates the perfect design and programming of the universal organizing principle and its essential continuation, the innate law, which is 100%/perfect and normal (Prin. 1, 20, 22, 27) by a 100%/perfect universal intelligence (Prin. 5). It is through the innate control that the standard of normal is established since the innate law is always normal and its function is always normal (Prin. 27).

ART. 107. ABNORMAL CYCLES (FLOWCHARTS)

Abnormal cycles are those in which the normal sequencing of processes of the normal flowchart cycle for coordination of activities is not within already established standards by the innate law. The cause in abnormal cycles is the cause of in-coordination of action. In the body, the causes of being outside the "normal" can be genetic, hereditary, environmental disruptions, vertebral subluxations or many others. Ultimately, it is due to the limitation of E/matter and time (Prin. 6). Chiropractic addresses exclusively the location, analysis, and the facilitation of the correction of vertebral subluxations for the restoration in transmission of the innate impulses through the practice of its objective.

ART. 108. COMPOUND OR COMPLEX CYCLES (FLOWCHARTS)

A compound flowchart is the combination of two cycles that are interoperable and process together simultaneously with coherence; the two cycles are dependent upon each other.

A complex flowchart is two or more cycles (up to billions) combined that are interoperable and process together simultaneously with coherence; those multiple cycles are dependent upon each other.

Compound and complex flowcharts must all have interoperability and coherence of all their processes so there can be normality and harmonious coordination of activities of all the parts of the body and proper soundness of the tissue cells for use in the body (Prin. 23). They are essential for different systems to work through dependence with each other with coherent harmonious actions.

These cycles (flowcharts) involve different levels of organization of living E/matter that manifest infinite motions from their design, programming of adjustability through error correction and restoration under innate processing. Adjustability leads to adaptation through reorganization from the innate law as living E/matter interacts with environmental circumstances. Adaptation of the organism can then, passed on through reproduction that includes genetic and hereditary transference. These different manifestations of organizational levels of E/matter are controlled by the innate law, that is an essential continuous extension of the universal organizing principle designed, and programmed by a universal intelligence processing to adapt the complexities of living E/matter to maintain the body alive for its lifespan if it is possible according to universal laws.

We refer to these different levels of organization as cellular organization, organ organization, system organization, and body organization. Since organization bespeaks intelligence, these vital processes are best described by different description of the function of the organizing principle, which is to organize information/F (Prin. 8) in the same way that we differently characterize non-living and living E/matter. From the perspective of the organizing principle, it is the same. From the living E/matter perspective, there are organizational differences, such as a butterfly has different organization than a baseball. Correspondingly there is a different organizational level between neurons and the skeletal system.

We should train ourselves to think and to visualize more than one cycle processing at the same time and remember that the infinite number of cycles is under the same innate control for all the tissue cells of the body. It is the innate law through its instantaneous integral adaptation that controls and governs the harmonious coherence of the infinite multitude of cycles within the body according to universal laws (Prin. 23, 24).

The following are flowcharts of cycles of continual systematic change of multiple cellular functions simultaneously interoperating under the innate control, though simplified. Please note that billions of these cycles are interacting moment by moment.

Dr. Claude Lessard

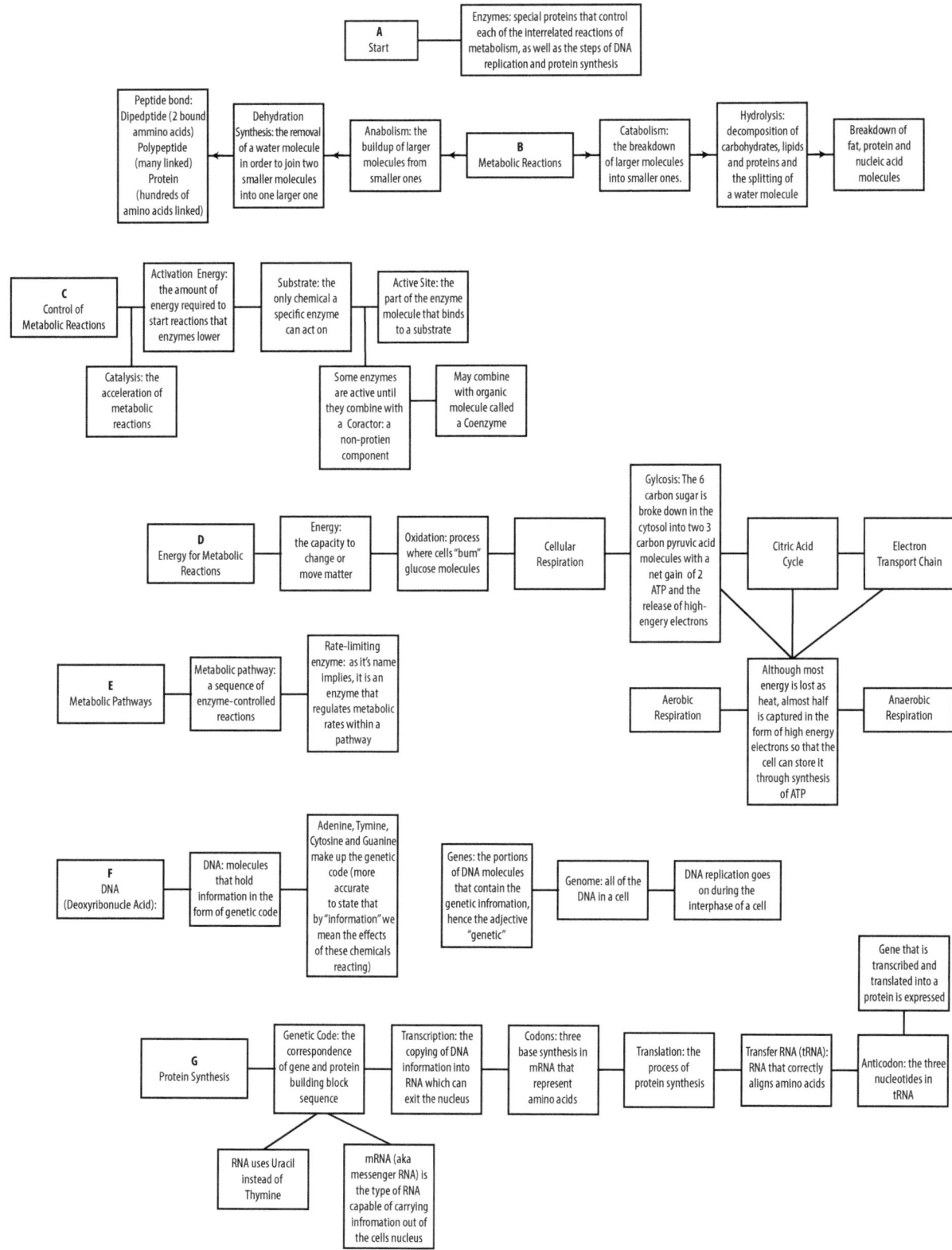

Fig. 13. One of many flow charts of continual, simultaneous, systematic change of multiple cellular functions processed by the innate law.

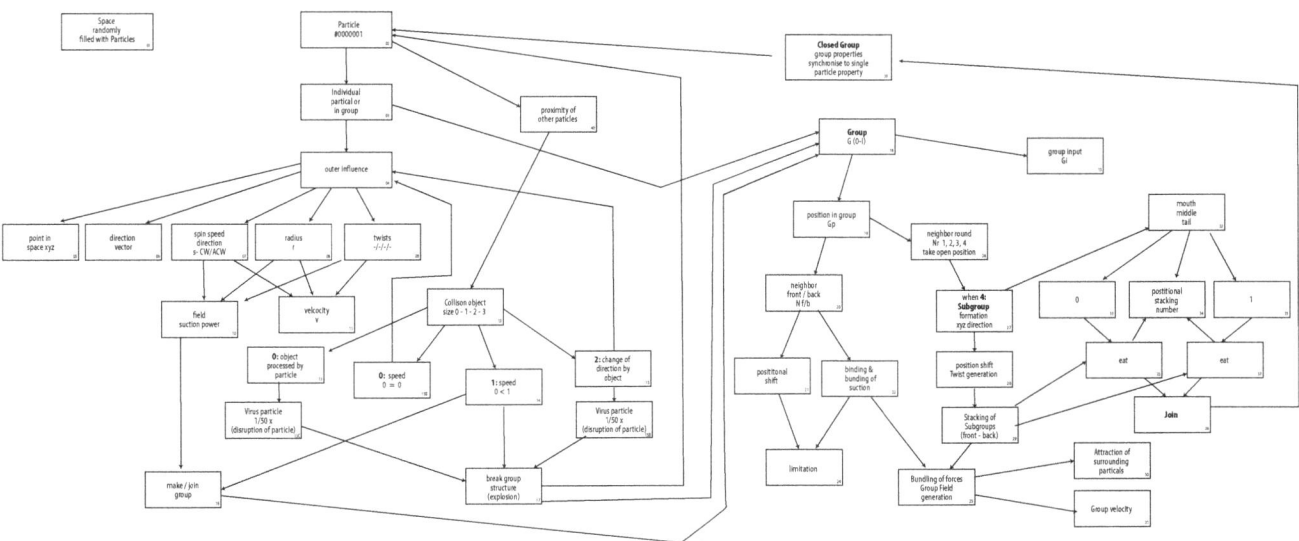

Fig. 14. An example of possible complex flowchart of cycles involving several interoperable cycles simultaneously.

ART. 109. SPECIAL SENSE CYCLE (FLOWCHART)

A special sense cycle consists of the many processes materializing between the special sense organ as periphery and the brain cells as center, and back again to periphery. In each, the cause is in the organized information/F of the periphery or the environment contingent on start point. The names of the special senses are: sight, hearing, smell, taste and touch.

The subject of special senses will be studied in further detail in Volume 4, and for that reason only two special sense cycles will be addressed in Volume 2. The main purpose of this study is to demonstrate the amazing innate control that is simultaneously governing the infinite multitude of cycles within the human body. Chiropractic addresses only the transmission of innate impulses through the practice of its objective.

The student should know that afferent general sense, as described in the normal complete cycle for coordination of activities, is not the same as the cycle studied in the afferent special sense cycle. The former relates to the processes concerning coordination of activities of all the parts of the body for coherence moment by moment, while the latter relates to the body's attempt to innately adapt to the external environment through sensory functions. There are multitude of assorted cycles operating between brain and periphery.

ART. 110. THE CYCLE OF SIGHT

The cycle of sight is the explanation of the process of sight, from the organ of sight (eye) as input sensor, to the processing organ (brain) as CPU and back again to periphery; all of these processes are under the governance of the universal organizing principle and its essential continuous extension, the innate law. The organs of sight have specialized nerve cells, whose special function is sensory. They are called sensory nerves and their purpose is to register the subtle vibration of light. The flowchart cycle illustrated here starts with the origin of light in the environment through the universal organizing principle. Since it is a complex cycle, three flowcharts are shown here to demonstrate the many processes involved. The cycle of sight, the normal complete cycle for coordination of activities, and the metabolism cycle of tissue cell. The three cycles operate simultaneously in coordination with each other.

Dr. Claude Lessard

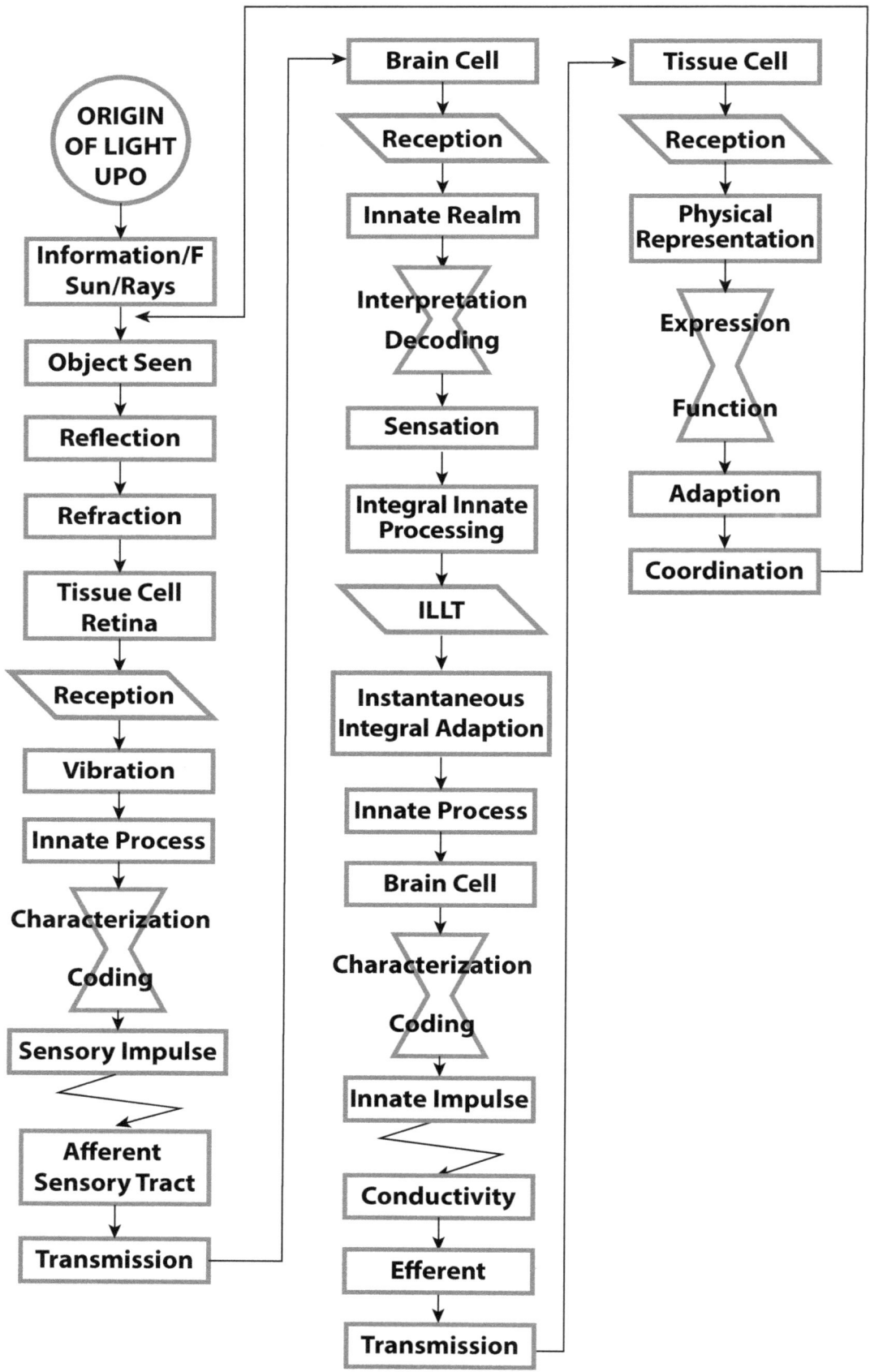

Fig. 15 a.

The 2027 Chiropractic Textbook Volume 2

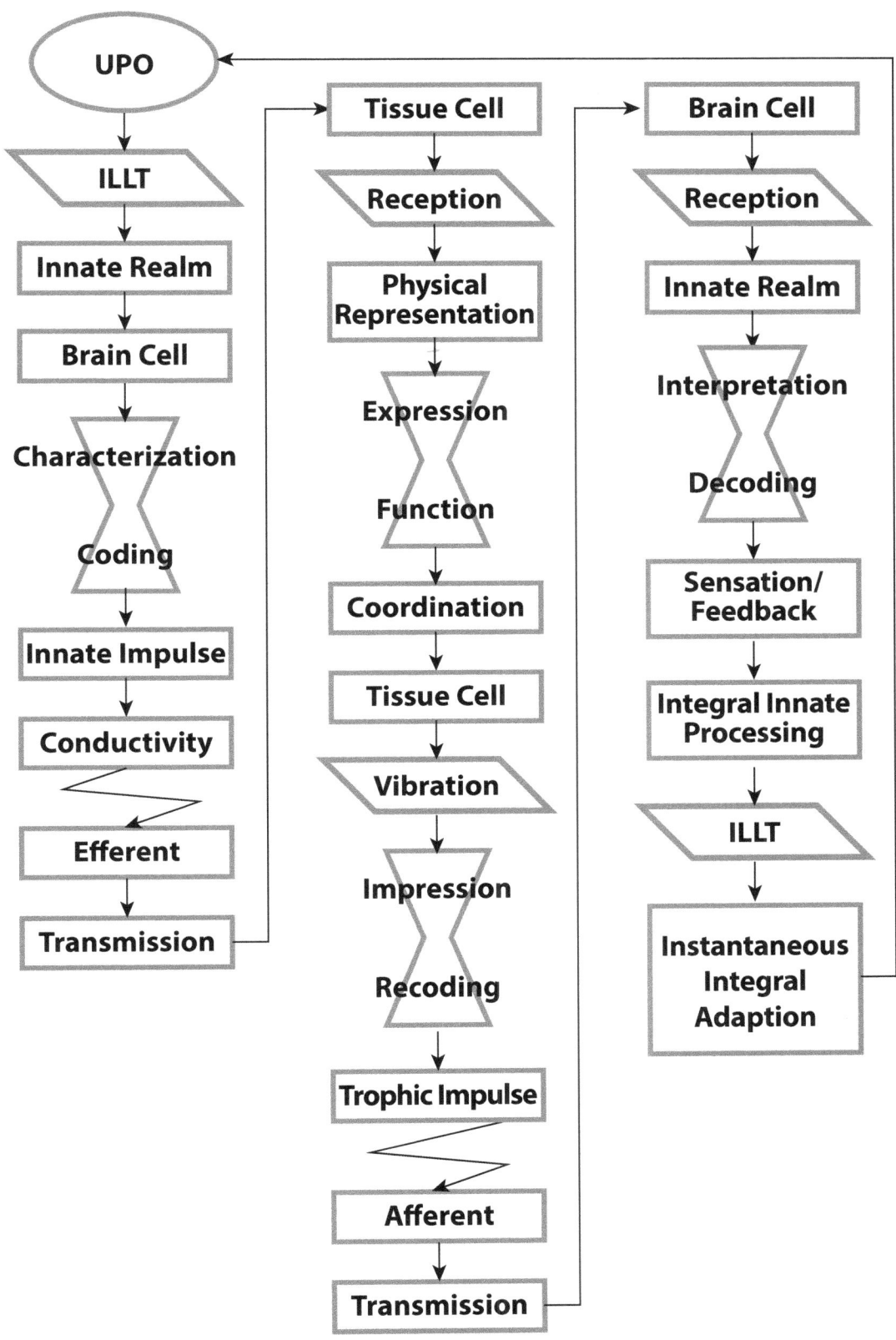

Fig. 15 b.

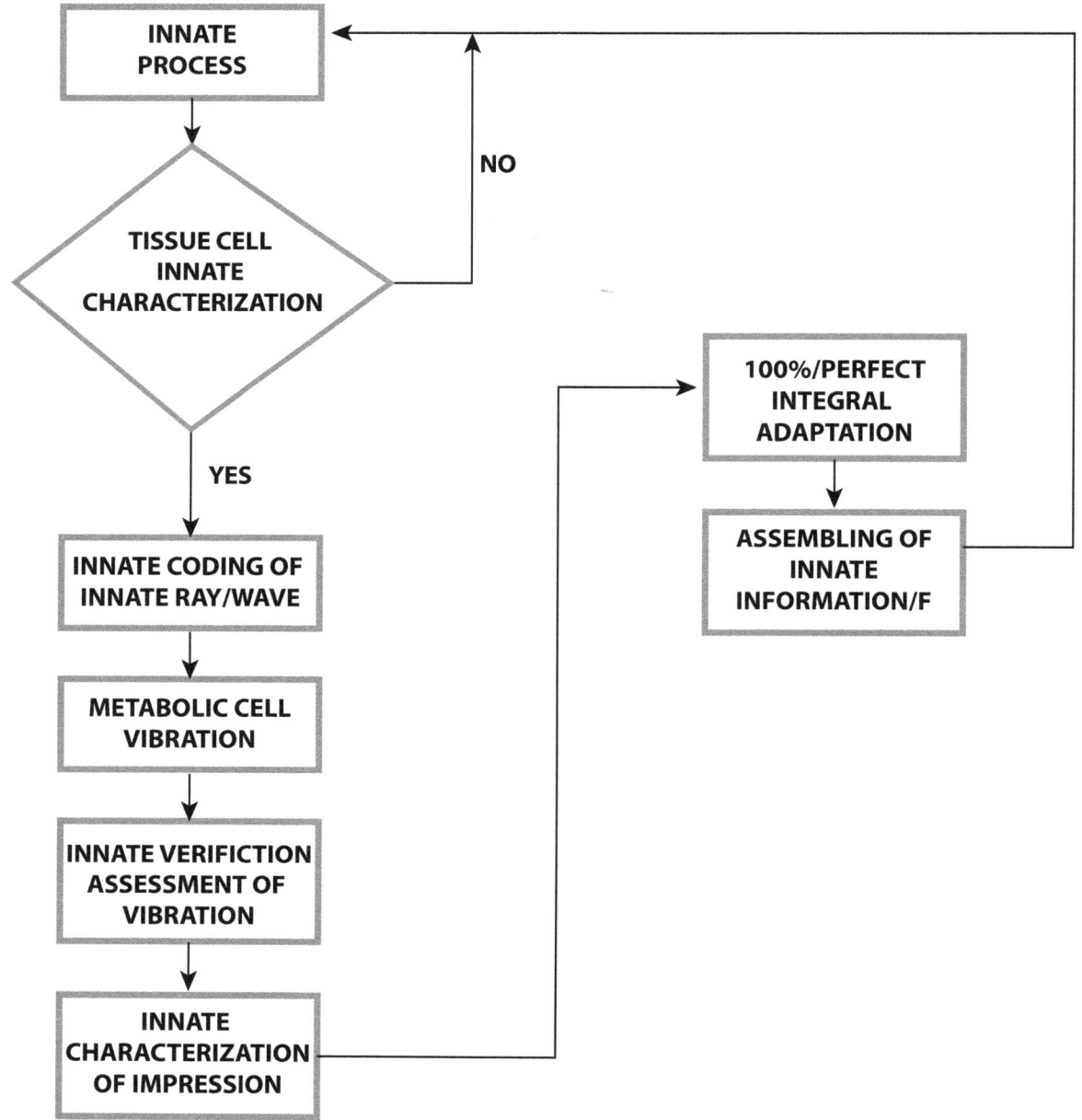

Fig. 15 c.

Fig. 15. Three flowcharts illustrating the cycle of sight that is a part of a complex cycle, including, (a)- Special sense of sight cycle in order to see and to adapt to the external environment under the innate control. (b)- Normal complete cycle for coordination of activities of all the parts of the body is the functional cycle under the innate control. (c)- Metabolism cycle of all tissue cells keeping the cells alive under the innate control.

These three cycles, along with the body chemistry circulation (shown in Fig. 26), are operating simultaneously within the organ of sight (eye) in this illustration. It is important to note that an entire multitude of cycles in the living body are operating simultaneously and coordinately under the 100%/perfect innate control moment by moment.

Light is in the form of an elementary discrete particle called photons. Light is information/F in the form of electromagnetic radiation of any wavelength. These photons are maintained in existence by the universal principle of organization. Light travels through the electromagnetic field of space/time and when it reaches the eye, it is refracted through the lens and contacts the retina. Within the retina are the specially constructed photo sensitive nerve cells that include rods and cones that are capable to register information/F vibrations of this kind. They function as the immediate instrument of sight by receiving the information/F. From there the impressions of vibrations, as sensory impulses, are transmitted over a special afferent sensory tract (optic nerve) to the brain for central processing. Once there, they are received and decoded for interpretation. Then from one unit of impression is derived one unit of sensation. This is the sensation of light. From the sensation of light through innate process, the innate decoding of the sensory impulse differentiates between primary (direct light) or secondary rays (reflected light from an object). Through integral innate processing the computed relationship with this object from the external environment is perfectly actualized. For the body to adapt to this environmental element, the innate control within the innate field assembles information/F from the inexhaustible supply of the universal principle of organization and characterizes them. It is through instantaneous integral adaptation by the innate law that coherent innate processes of relationships between internal and external environment become balanced. Within the brain (CPU), characterization of innate impulses, conducted through efferent nerves to the tissue cell for physical representation, is computed to express information/F, by the motion the body part, for the sake of coordination of activities. In the sight cycle, the cell-sensors of the eye are basically sensing electromagnetic waves, which is universal information/F from the external environment as they contact the eye striking the retina. Universal information/F is then immediately adapted and coded into innate information/F to be transmitted to the brain for central processing and decoding. The afferent transmission of sensory impulses of special sense organs is different than the afferent transmission of the feedback trophic impulses/signals, of body parts, for coordination of activities of the normal complete cycle. Sensory impulses are for environmental innate adaptation. Feedback trophic impulses/signals, of body parts, are for the coordination of their activities.

Dr. Claude Lessard

REVIEW QUESTIONS FOR ARTICLES 103 - 110

1. What is a chiropractic cycle?
2. What is a compound cycle?
3. What is a complex cycle?
4. Where or what should the origin point of reasoning be in a chiropractic cycle?
5. What is the cause of the normal complete cycle for coordination of activities?
6. What is the cause of the normal special sense cycle?
7. Specific to chiropractic, what is the cause in abnormal cycles?
8. Specific to chiropractic, what is the cause in restoration cycles?
9. What is the general cause of the maintaining the existence of all things in the universe?
10. Name the physiological cycles in the body.
11. What is the normal cycle?
12. What is the abnormal cycle?
13. What is the cause of the cycle of sight?
14. Why are flowcharts instruments of the organizing principle?

ART. 111. ABNORMAL SPECIAL SENSE CYCLE (FLOWCHART)

A special sense cycle can be made abnormal by interference to sensory nerves. Any interference with the transmission of innate information/F in the body can affect the sense cycle and render it abnormal due to chemical imbalance or tissue cell replication. Chiropractic only addresses interference with transmission of innate impulses caused by vertebral subluxations *(See Fig. 15, 18)*.

ART. 112. INTER-FIELD CYCLE (FLOWCHART)

A complex cycle deals with the universal field, the innate field, and the educated field within the body. They are fields of operations. They are what we call operating systems. Those three fields are arbitrary and they are non-discrete, non-material, and they relate to different levels of complexity of organized E/matter. They are in union with the material. In reality, there is only one unified field within space/time, and within it, is contained unlimited information/F of multiple fields that unite the organizing principle and E/matter. Cycles describe the processes of the union of organizing principle and E/matter of the universe, including the living E/matter of the human body. The complexity of the interoperability of a multitude of cycles baffles the human mind. It underscores the importance of restoration of the interconnectivity of all the body parts through the correction of vertebral subluxations.

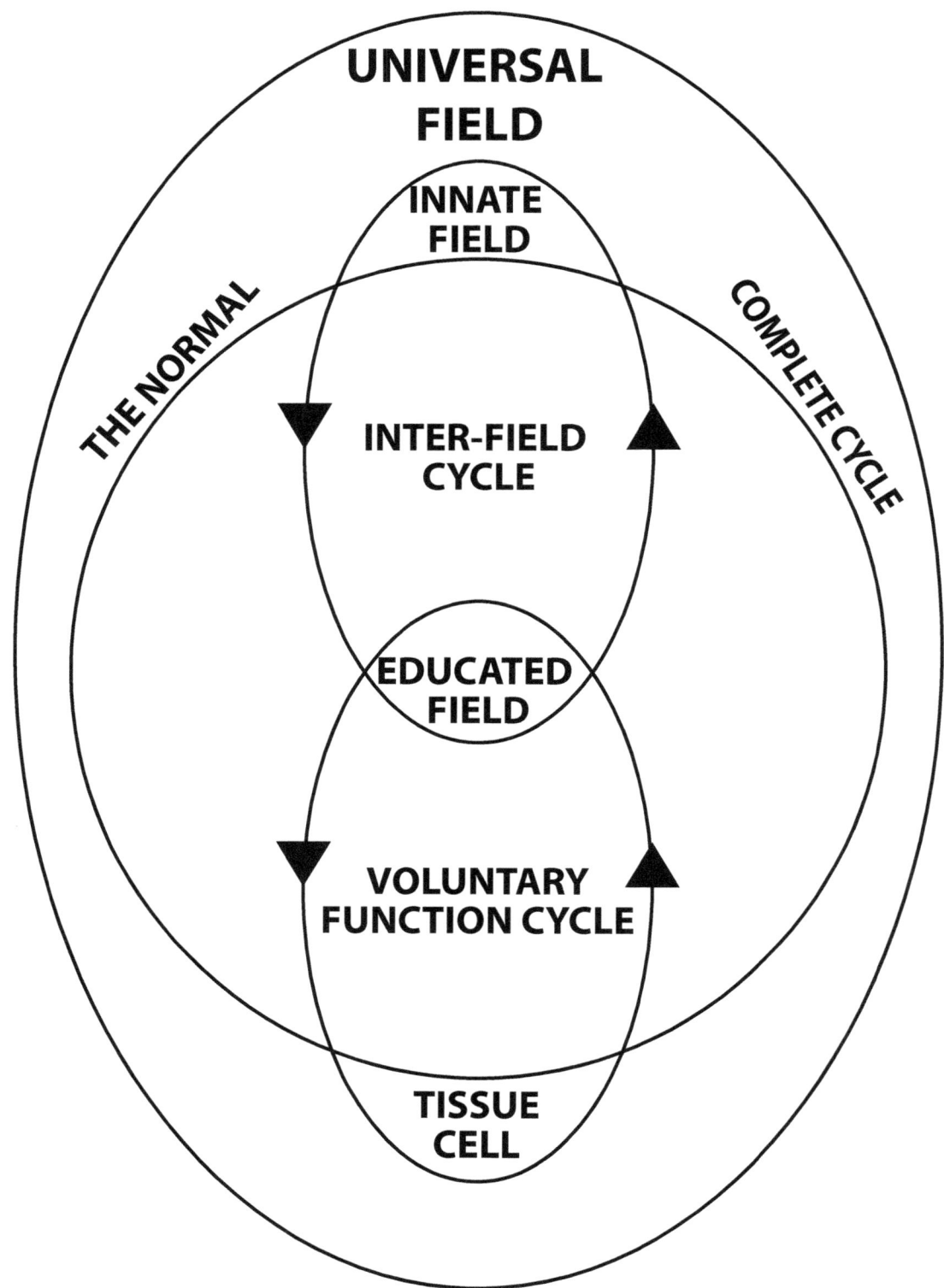

Fig. 16. A complex cycle diagram shows the relationship between the universal field, the innate field and the educated field. The student should note that the universal field is where the universal principle of organization operates to maintain all of E/matter in existence. The universal field is everywhere and it is a continual operating system of the universal principle of organization (Prin. 1).

ART. 113. THE UNIVERSAL DIAGRAM OF CYCLES (FLOWCHARTS)

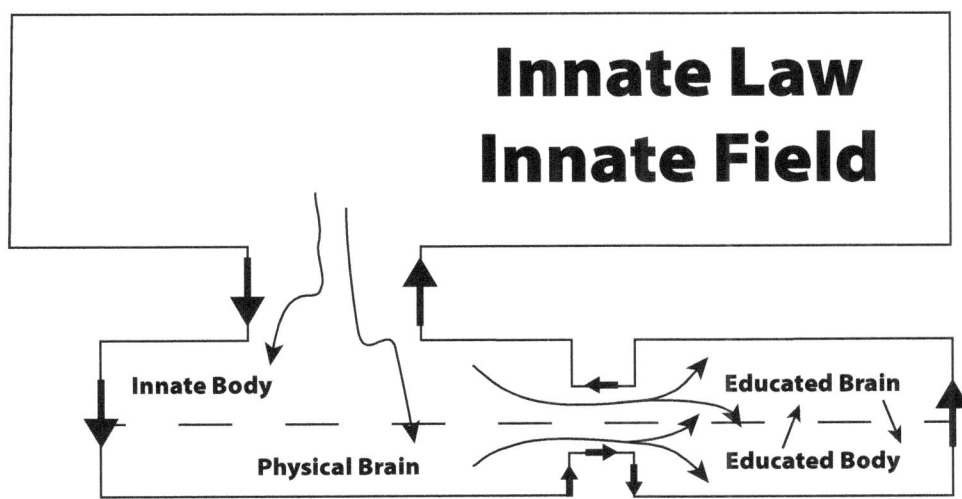

Fig. 17. Illustates the relationships of all cycles. It is a combination of Fig. 5 and Fig. 9 from Volume 1. This diagram demonstrates that, for coordination of activities, the course of innate information/F is followed around the borderline the diagram as shown by the arrows around the diagram. For cell metabolism, the course of information/F is within the diagram as shown by the waves inside the diagram. Special senses cycle and voluntary actions cycle are also following the arrows around the borderline. The universal diagram of cycles is a complex cycle that includes all the multitude of cycles in the body that operate simultaneously.

As one traces the borderline arrows, for coordination of activities, notice that information/F is synchronized and processed step by step. From physical brain (that is also part of innate body) innate impulses coordinate the activities of the innate body. Then passing through educated brain some innate impulses are modified (tinctured) into educated impulses for the voluntary actions using the educated body. Progressing through trophic impulses/signals feedback, the loop returns to the physical brain through the innate field for instantaneous integral adaptation in order to coordinate the actions of all the parts of the body. Following the waved arrows within the diagram, since every cell of the body are innate body, we notice that they are supplied with information/F from within each cell for their specific metabolism moment by moment. The educated brain and the educated body are also part of the innate body. The feedback loop is then completed through the same cycles as it informs the state of the soundness of the cell from its state of coordination of function. If the soundness of the cell is innate-normal and there is no interference in transmission of innate impulses, there will be coordination of activities. If either the cell is unsound or there is interference in transmission of innate impulses, then there will be not be coordination of activities. This is determined through instantaneous integral adaptation under the innate control. Chiropractic addresses only interference with transmission of innate impulses caused directly or indirectly by vertebral subluxations (Prin. 31a). This diagram can be applied to various cycles, including the simple, compound, and complex cycles.

ART. 114. A WRITTEN DIAGRAM SHOWING INNATE AND EDUCATED REALM

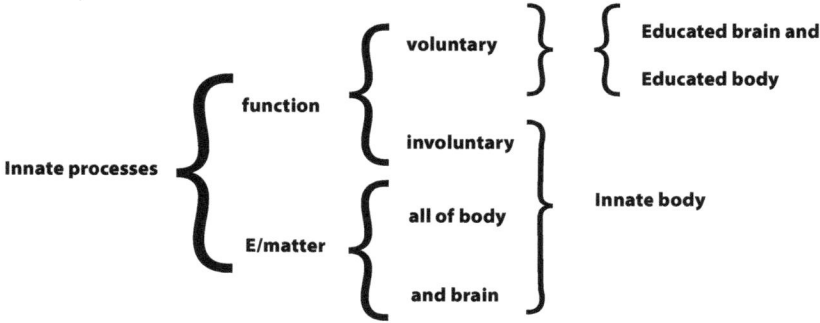

An alternate way of viewing Fig. 17.

All processes of the body are under the innate control from the innate realm regarding the involuntary function of living E/matter since all E/matter is innate body. Educated control from the educated realm affects and modifies (tinctures) some innate impulses passing through the educated brain for the voluntary functions of educated body.

ART. 115. THE VERTEMERE CYCLE (FLOWCHART)

The vertemere cycle is the cycle from the brain to the tissues, holding in situ the vertebra in question. A vertebral subluxation that is affecting a nerve from brain to organ also affects the neurons supplying its own tissues, and that is why it exists as a vertebral subluxation.

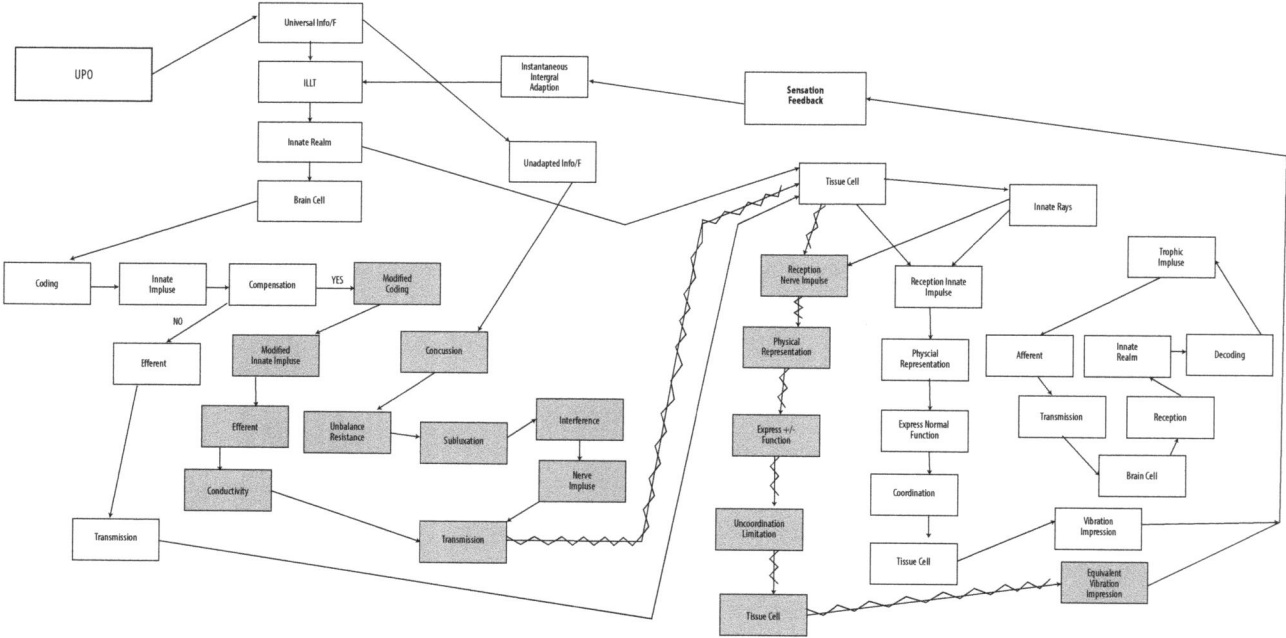

Fig. 18. Normal complete cycle for coordination of activities compounded with the vertemere cycle showing a concussion of information/F where non-adapted external invasive information/F overcomes the internal innate natural genetic resistance of the body that causes a vertebral subluxation interfering with transmission of innate impulses (Prin. 29, 30, 31a). It introduces an abnormal cycle of in-coordination of activities at the vertemere.

Within the flowchart of Fig. 18, the clear boxes represent the normal complete cycles for coordination of activities, the dark boxes represent a cycle from brain cell to the tissue cells of the vertemere, which is the region of the vertebra itself. It demonstrates the unbalanced resistance resulting from a concussion of information/F. This makes it a compound cycle for study. This is one of the most important cycles in the study of chiropractic, and the students should make themselves well-acquainted with it. It is the only cycle with immediate practical application, and it is the basis for the art of chiropractic technique, which will be discussed in Volume 4.

This flowchart explains the basis for the vertebral subluxation and why it does not correct itself in spite of the computation of information/F under the innate control. The interference with the transmission of innate impulses to the tissues of the vertemere limits the processing of a vertebral adjustment by the innate processes that would be using the vertebral muscles to move the articular facets of the vertebra within its normal juxtaposition. Fig. 18 demonstrates the in-coordination of the abnormal vertemere cycle due to the vertebral subluxation. Even though the innate processes are computing all information/F available, they cannot restore the vertebra to it proper juxtaposition due to the lack of or incorrect information/F transmitted to the vertemere. This means that the innate law is continually adapting information/F in order to process a vertebral adjustment. If we could analyze the state of the vertemere through muscle palpation, identifying the working muscles and their corrective vectors, we could introduce an adjustic thrust (Fig. 20), which would provide the added information/F necessary to be adapted by the innate law to process a vertebral adjustment (Prin. 31a, 31b). This is the basis for ADIO analysis. In the 1970s ADIO analysis was founded by Reggie Gold, D.C.. We co-developed the ADIO analysis in order to determine the location and the corrective vectors of the working muscles of the subluxated vertebra. Reproductions of a few articles published in the early 1980s addressing ADIO analysis will be provided in Volume 4. Please note, that the arrow going from the innate realm directly to the tissue cell indicates the adaptation of the tissue cell for metabolism through innate rays/waves. Innate rays/waves are not addressed by chiropractic. Chiropractic only addresses interference of innate impulses from vertebral subluxations.

ART. 116. UNIVERSAL INFORMATION/F

Synonyms: External information/F, environmental information/F, physical information/F, chemical information/F.

Universal information/F is the generalized information/F of the universe which obey universal laws, and is not adapted for useful purposes (Prin. 11). However, it absolutely can be adapted and characterized (coded) for useful purposes, especially in the body following the law of adaptation according to universal laws (Prin. 23, 24, 25, 26). If it is adapted in the body, it is beneficial to the body (constructive); if it is not adapted in the body, it is harmful to the body (deconstructive). It may be applied either inside or outside of the body. Some universal information/F is always inside the body, as it cannot be kept out (Prin. 1, 16). If the body is innate-normal, it is always adapted, when it is inside the body. It may affect the body in numerous ways as physical, chemical, emotional, technical, or mechanical ramifications.

Universal information/F has already been described in Volume 1. It is necessary to the body to maintain universal balance and to maintain E/matter in existence, so that the innate law intrinsic to the body of the living thing will have some dynamic information/F to adapt, control and govern. It should be understood that the body experiences universal information/F in necessary circumstances, as well as harmful ones. We know them as incidents, weather, food, drink, sunlight, and a myriad of others. Sometimes it is harmful, as accidents, inclement weather, poison, pollution, stress, etc. Interestingly enough, stress is an interaction between information/F and the internal resistance to counter in order to keep the body in balance. It was Hans Seyle who incorporated the term "stress" in 1956, following his 1936 seminal work.[26] It is quite obvious to see that the cause of vertebral subluxation is a concussion of information/F where the external invasion overcomes the internal resistance. We know that vertebral subluxations are always harmful to the body (Prin. 30, 31a).

ART. 117. INVASIVE INFORMATION/F

Invasive information/F are universal and produce their effects upon tissue. The innate law can adapt them for use in the body and for the coordination of all the parts of the body for mutual benefit (Prin. 23) as long as they do not overcome the internal resistance for balance. If the body needs to resist them to keep balance, the innate computation will process accordingly. If, however, the invasion overcomes the natural genetic resistance of the body, a vertebral subluxation will occur and the resistance will be lowered due to the limitation of E/matter, which is increased (worsened) by the vertebral subluxation.

Invasive information/F is physical or chemical and may not good or bad. However, if the invasive information/F overcomes the internal resistance of the body, then it is not adapted by the innate law, due to the limitations of E/matter, and it acts in an un-adapted way, meaning deconstructive toward structural E/matter (Prin. 26). It comes in numerous forms whether physical or chemical and it basically participates in the cause of vertebral subluxations when it is not adapted by the innate law.

Invasive information/F is well known. We fail to acknowledge some of it because some of it is insidious. It may enter the body as chemical and if not adapted, will begin their deconstructive work toward structural E/matter (Prin. 26), or it may call for very violent adaptation. The information/F of extreme weather, heat, cold, etc., call upon the material resources of the ability of the educated brain to use and the innate control for severe adaptation. If the internal resistance of the body is low, some drastic information/F can do harm. Not all invasive information/F provokes violent resistance while it is adapted by the innate law and it does not cause any problems. On the contrary, it becomes the source of constructive survival values for the life of the body.

ART. 118. INNATE INFORMATION/F

Universal information/F adapted and organized by innate control through innate computation and processing in the body is innate information/F. It is universal information/F adapted and assembled for dynamic functional processes of capability for use in the body and coordination of action of all its parts (Prin. 23). Innate information/F causes tissue cells to function in order to relate to the internal and external environment of the body. Innate information/F may be for adaptation to other universal information/F, which have not been adapted in order to balance, annul, check, transform, characterize, or otherwise adapt it.

ART. 119. INTERNAL RESISTANCE

The internal resistance is actualized through the adaption of information/F by the innate law that is computing and organizing it to counteract un-adapted invasive information/F in order to keep the body in balance. The manifestation of the information/F of the internal resistance comes in numerous forms whether physical or chemical or other stressors-related. Examples of manifestations in physical forms are

---

26. Selye, H. "The Stress of Life." New York: McGraw-Hill Book Company, Inc. (1956) p.1

movement of tissue cells, such as in chemical forms are antidotes, oxidation, etc., or in stress forms like sudden reflex motion as the knee jerk reflex.

When there is unbalanced information/F (non-adapted) within the body it is deconstructive toward structural E/matter (Prin. 26), often causing a vertebral subluxation. When there is the presence of unbalanced information/F, it is never due to a lack from the 100%/perfect innate law (Prin. 22) but it is always due to the limitation of E/matter (Prin. 24). If it becomes adapted under the innate control, it becomes constructive toward structural E/matter (Prin. 26) and may be combined with others for resistance purposes.

Regarding the adjustic thrust, it is an external educated universal information/F and it may either be adapted by the innate law to produce a vertebral adjustment, or it may be resisted, under the innate control, to keep the body from being harmed by the useless move. If the adjustic thrust overcomes the internal resistance of the body, it will participate in causing a vertebral subluxation. The internal resistance of the body under the innate control will always counteract invading information/F if it is not beyond the limits of adaptability of the tissues (Prin. 23, 24); otherwise, a concussion of information/F will occur and a vertebral subluxation will ensue (Prin. 31a). The student must always remember that chiropractic is only about what is possible according to universal laws (Prin. 24). An improper adjustic thrust may cause a vertebral subluxation if it overpowers the internal resistance of the body.

ART. 120. TRAUMA

Trauma is injury to the tissue cells due to an accident or poisoning. In trauma the tissue cells are not necessarily un-coordinated and if transmission of innate impulse remains normal, healing will quickly occur through cellular replacement. The tissue cells may not be completely sound when injured. However, the relationship between coordination of activities and this traumatic condition will, if there is no interference with transmission of innate impulses, continue to allow the injured tissue cells to still participate, through cellular replacement, within their limitations, in the coordination of the body part involved. Here is a distinction that may help. In trauma, the tissue cells are still "clear" if they receive normal transmission of innate impulses and they have proper metabolism. It is when the tissue cells do not receive normal transmission of innate impulses and/or lack proper metabolism that they are not "clear", and are un-coordinated.

Trauma is in the field of surgery, and a chiropractor would have no work to do in this case, unless there is a vertebral subluxation, causing interference with the transmission of innate impulses. Trauma itself may produce a concussion, where external invasion overcomes internal resistance thus causing a vertebral subluxation. Depending on the number of cells that have been traumatized, when there is normal transmission of innate impulses to the body part, and with proper metabolism, cellular replacement will, in time, regenerate the tissue cells of that body part. If the trauma is too extensive, regeneration may never take place.

ART. 121. DISEASE AND DIS-EASE

Disease is a term used by physicians for sickness. To them it is an entity and is worthy of a name, hence diagnosis. DIS-EASE is a chiropractic term meaning not having ease; or lack of ease (The term DIS-EASE should always be capitalized and hyphenated). It is then a lack of entity. It is a condition of E/matter when it does not have the property of ease. Ease is the entity, and DIS-EASE is the lack of entity. In chiropractic it pertains more specifically to the lack of ease of the neuron-transmitters that are interfered with vertebral subluxations. DIS-EASE leads to incoordination of activities of the parts of the body (Prin. 29, 30, 31a, 32). Principle 31 states: Interference with transmission of conducted innate information/force causes incoordination of DIS-EASE.

DIS-EASE, in chiropractic, is indicative of the body being minus something that should be restored in order to make it innate-normal. What is this minus something that should be restored to innate-normal in the body? It is normal transmission of innate impulses (Prin. 27, 29). The lack of ease occurs at the site of the interference of the neurons from the vertebral subluxation. It is a condition of the transmitting E/matter that does not have the property of ease. DIS-EASE is a non-entity. Ease is the entity. The cause of the lack of ease of the neuron-transmitters is what needs to be corrected in the body. Chiropractic restores the momentum of transmission of innate impulses, back to innate-normal (Prin. 27) for coordination of activities through the facilitation of the correction of vertebral subluxations (Prin. 30, 31a, 31b, 32). The aim of chiropractic is to restore, to innate-normal, the momentum of the transmission of innate impulses. If restoration of the momentum of transmission of innate impulses does not take place, this lack of ease (DIS-EASE) of the transmitting E/matter will then lead to incoordination of activities of body parts (Prin. 29, 30, 31a, 32).

Regarding trauma, the tissues are not degenerated or depleted. They are just injured. Sometimes a wound will regenerate readily through cellular replacement under the innate control if the whole body is receiving innate-normal transmission of innate impulses and has sound metabolism (Prin. 23).

DIS-EASE is the condition of the transmitting E/matter that does not have the property of ease. This lack of ease of the neuron-transmitters interferes with the momentum of transmission of innate impulses and always leads to in-coordination of activities in the whole body (Prin. 30, 32). Chiropractic addresses the vertebral subluxation, which is the cause of DIS-EASE (Prin. 30, 31a). When there is no interference in transmission of innate impulses, there is a continuous supply and computation from the innate law (Prin. 33) to ensure coordination of action of all the parts of the body in fulfilling their roles and purposes (Prin. 32), if it is possible according to universal laws (Prin. 24). What comes as a result of in-coordination of activities is of no concern to the chiropractor because it simply means that the limitations of E/matter has been made worse by the vertebral subluxation The only concern of the chiropractor is the restoration of the momentum of transmission of innate impulses to innate-normal through the practice of the chiropractic objective based on the 33 principles of its basic science. Limitations of E/matter is a medical issue and is not within the purview of chiropractic.

The principle of coordination within the body must be satisfied for continuous coherent actions of all body parts in fulfilling their roles and purposes (Prin. 32) and it must come from within through the restoration of the momentum of transmission of innate impulses (Prin. 29, 30, 31a, 31b), by the location, analysis, and the facilitation of the correction of vertebral subluxations.

REVIEW QUESTIONS FOR ARTICLES 111 - 121

1. Provide three ways in which special sense can be made abnormal.
2. In the inter-field cycle, what tissue is "periphery?"
3. What cycle has the most practical application?
4. Why does a misplaced vertebra, which is subluxated, remains a vertebral subluxation?
5. Where is "periphery" in the vertemere cycle?
6. What is the character of universal information/F?
7. Is universal information/F applied inside or outside the body?
8. What is invasive information/F?
9. Is invasive information/F synonymous with universal information/F?
10. What is innate information/F?
11. What is the internal resistance of the body?
12. Is the internal resistance of the body synonymous with innate information/F or is it a specific class of innate information/F?
13. When the information/F of the internal resistance of the body are "out of timing" or unbalanced, what are they apt to produce?
14. What is the cause of the internal resistance of the body to be "out of timing" or unbalanced?
15. What is trauma?
16. What is disease?
17. What is DIS-EASE?
18. What is the distinction between trauma and in-coordination?
19. Regarding incoordination of DIS-EASE what is the sole aim of chiropractic?

ART. 122. THE CAUSE OF INCOORDINATION *OF* DIS-EASE

The cause of INCOORDINATION *OF* DIS-EASE is interference in the transmission of innate impulses. The vertebral subluxation is the physical representation of the cause of the lack of ease of the transmitting E/matter. It must be remembered, as we saw in the previous article, that it is the impingement upon the neurons, which interfere with the transmission of conducted information/F in the neurons that causes them to lack ease and become unable to normally transmit innate impulses with innate-normal momentum (Prin. 27, 28, 29, 31). It is only the transmitting E/matter that can be in a state of DIS-EASE as the cause of incoordination of activities. It is DIS-EASE that leads to in-coordination of action of the body parts, thus violating the principle of coordination (Prin. 32).

ART. 123. HOW THE CAUSE CAUSES INCORDINATION *OF* DIS-EASE

Interference with the momentum of transmission of innate impulses causes INCOORDINATION *OF* DIS-EASE of the whole body by preventing the tissue cells of the body part to receive the intended instruction from the innate impulses in a timely manner (Prin. 6). The body part becomes uncoordinated in its activities due to an increase of the limitations of its E/matter and therefore lacks adaptability (Prin. 24). If there is interference with the conducted innate impulses, there is a lack of adaptation of the body part, which is due to the further increase of limitation of E/matter of the whole body. This means that if a body part is uncoordinated, the principle of coordination is violated and thus the whole body becomes uncoordinated in its activities. The character of the innate impulse has reverted back to an un-adapted universal information/F from a change in the momentum in transmission. Lack of adaptation means that universal information/F will work uncontrolled. Un-adapted universal information/F is deconstructive toward structural E/matter (Prin. 26). Therefore, the tissue cells of the body part will act un-coordinately. INCOORDINATION *OF* DIS-EASE is due to interference with the momentum of transmission of innate impulses (Prin. 29, 30). Chiropractic is about the restoration of the momentum of transmission of innate impulses, back to innate-normal, through the practice of its objective, which is based on the 33 principles of its basic science. According to chiropractic's basic science, a body free of vertebral subluxation, and with sound metabolism, satisfies the principle of coordination (Prin. 23, 31a, 31b, 32). Chiropractic is exclusively concerned with the facilitation of the correction of vertebral subluxation.

ART. 124. THE ABNORMAL COMPLETE CYCLE CAUSING IN-COORDINATION OF ACTIVITIES

The abnormal complete cycle resulting in incoordination of activities is a compound cycle consisting of the abnormal cycle from brain to part, combined with the abnormal cycle from brain to vertemere. The orderly sequence of steps within the flow chart has been broken simultaneously in both cycles.

The table of steps is given in Fig. 18. The student is not required to commit to memory the steps of the flowchart, but to be able to reason with the steps as guides in order to eventually obtain a working knowledge of this flowchart.

From the shaded boxes the nerve is no longer properly transmitting the innate impulses with normal momentum due to the concussion causing the vertebral subluxation. This nerve is now carrying a universal information/F in the form of a nerve impulse that is out of timing and it is not an innate impulse any longer. There is abnormal transmission at the impinged neurons along the course of the neuromere. When the nerve impulse, which is without the proper innate-normal transmission, reaches the tissue cell, its instructions may be received by an innate-normal tissue cell due to innate rays/waves that are providing for its metabolism. However, the traveling impulse is no longer a perfectly assembled innate information/F. At this point, it is practically a universal information/F and is basically a nerve impulse without innate constructive information/F, without momentum-direction. It is not what was coded from the instantaneous integral adaptation computed under the innate control for that specific moment. There will be abnormal physical representation. The normal tissue cell receiving the nerve impulse will not express the intended innate instructive information/F. At this point, the adaptability of the tissue of the body part is compromised (Prin. 18, 19, 24) and it will act without the intended innate instructions and thus will be deprived of what is necessary for proper coordination of activities (Prin. 32). Of course, the whole body will be affected because other body parts will eventually lack coordination of activities. The whole body takes on a degree of unsoundness and the non-cooperative actions of that body part's tissue will participate in the unsoundness of other tissue cells.

This now abnormal tissue cell is acting and expressing information/F corresponding to its character (function and soundness), which is called equivalent vibration. It is acting as manifestation of the body part. The composite information/F is collected by the afferent nerve and is normally transmitted by the afferent nerve as equivalent impressions constructed as trophic impulses/signals reaching the brain cell. Trophic impulses/signals are information/F that have been characterized by the innate law with specific modal impression of vibrations of the metabolic and coordinative state of a tissue cell as to whether it functions coordinately or not. A trophic impulse/signal is transmitted through afferent nerves, then waving its way through the innate field to be received by the brain cell (CPU) as feedback. It is processed for computation and interpretation of the equivalent vibrations giving equivalent sensations. This provides the exact true state of function, whether normal or abnormal, of the tissue cell for an equivalent integral processing for coordination of activities, since afferent nerves are not subject to interference in transmission from vertebral subluxation (Vol. 1, Fig. 1). Then it is ready for instantaneous integral adaptation by the innate law to proceed in order to make compensation to correct the vertebral subluxation to restore transmission of innate impulses for coordination of activities *(See Fig. 18)*. Observe that this cycle will continue until there is adequate adapted information/F to produce a vertebral adjustment. The adjustic thrust provides specific information/F with the further intent that it will be adapted and processed by the innate law in order to produce the vertebral adjustment, which is the exclusive concern of chiropractic *(See Fig. 20)*.

ART. 125. THE ABNORMAL SENSE CYCLE

An abnormal sense cycle is the result of direct interference with transmission of the sensory nerve, or indirectly by interference with transmission of innate impulses causing in-coordination of activities of distant parts of the body supplying necessary substances to the sensory nerve or the sensory organ itself through the serous circulation *(See Fig. 26)*. The sensory organ may not be sound or its innate impulses are interfered with by vertebral subluxation directly or indirectly in any other parts of the body that may affect the sensory organ. Regardless of the reason, chiropractic addresses exclusively the correction of vertebral subluxations. The physiological functions of the tissue cells of the body are not the concern of chiropractic. The aim of the chiropractor is to practice the chiropractic objective, which is the location, analysis, and facilitation of the correction of vertebral subluxation for an innate-normal transmission of innate impulses.

Dr. Claude Lessard

ART. 126. HOW TO APPLY THE NORMAL CYCLE FOR COORDINATION OF ACTIVITIES

Here is an example with a flow chart: The stomach cycle is necessary for coordination of activities of body. The stomach processes external information/F and E/matter in terms of inputs comprised of external foodstuff. Digestion, one of the nine numbered primary functions, is the function considered here for the purpose of understanding the importance of innate processing and computation, which is a function of the nutritional groups. This illustrates the amazing innate computation required under the innate control to adapt, process and govern the multitude of operational steps necessary for coordination of activities of every numberless cycles within the body simultaneously. Chiropractors participate in this amazing innate process when they practice the chiropractic objective, which is to locate, analyze, and facilitate the correction of vertebral subluxation for an innate-normal transmission of innate impulses.

Every organ, gland and system of the body has an organic function cycle for coordination of activities that operate simultaneously under the direct innate control of the innate law for a lifetime according to universal laws. It necessitates an innate-normal transmission of innate impulses to satisfy the principle of coordination (Prin. 32).

The 2027 Chiropractic Textbook Volume 2

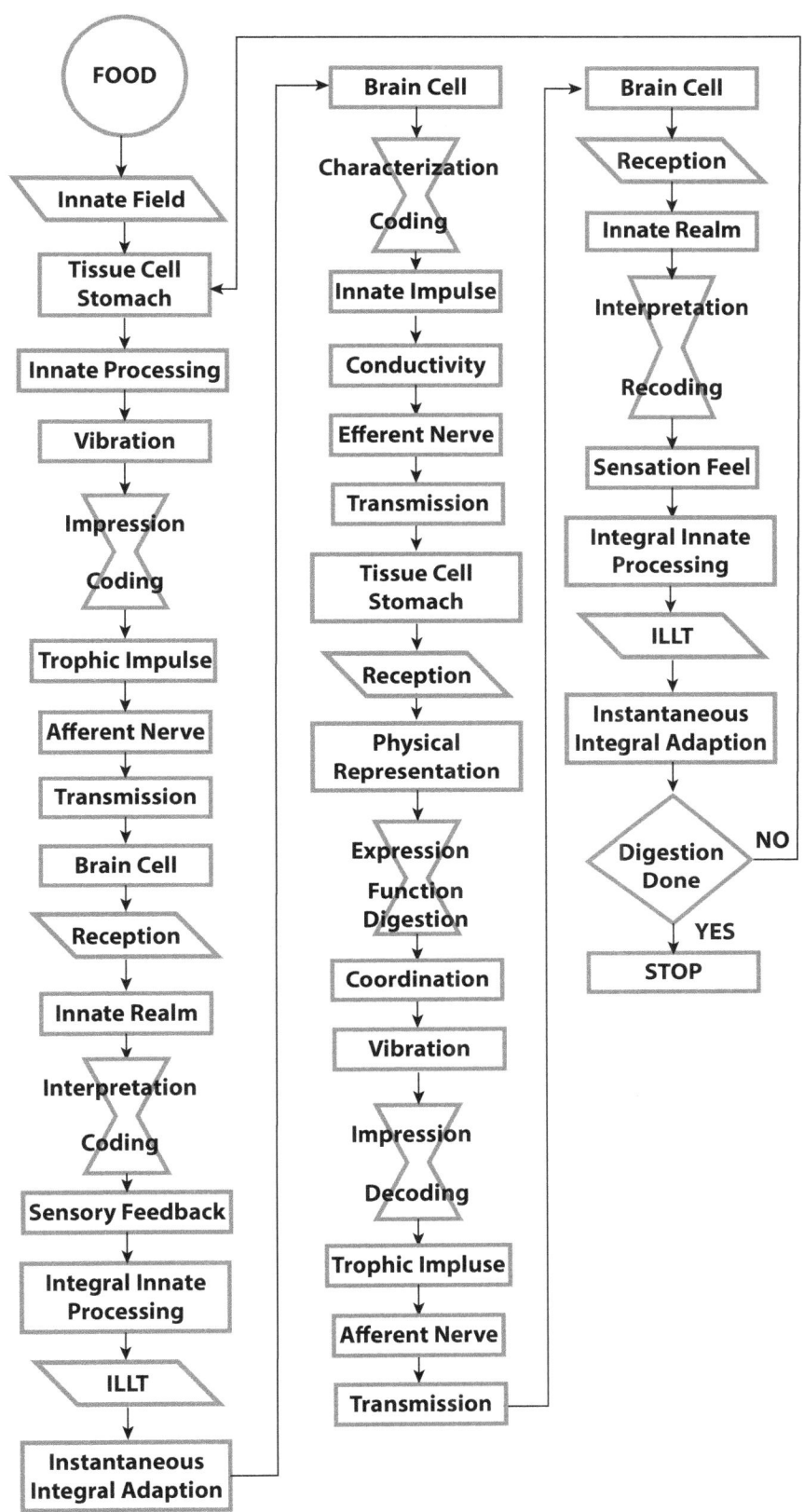

Fig. 19. Demonstrates a flow chart of a normal organic function cycle for coordination of activities. As an example the flowchart of the normal cycle of the function of the stomach as an organ is shown. The cycle is self-explanatory.

Dr. Claude Lessard

ART. 127. OTHER USE OF THE NORMAL CYCLE FOR COORDINATION OF ACTIVITIES

Special sense adaptation cycles explain the innate processing of external information/F received from the environment from the special senses. The student can use some of the flowcharts of Fig. 15a to demonstrate some of its steps. Notice that the first flowchart can be interfered by vertebral subluxations between steps of sensory impulse and afferent sensory tract. The student is reminded to not confuse it with the afferent nerve used to transmit the trophic impulse/signal which waves its afferent way through the innate field for coordination of activities, which cannot be interfered by vertebral subluxation because the cell body is outside the spinal cord *(See Fig. 1)*. Furthermore, the feedback for coordination of activities must be always true.

Special sense organs are literally sensors that receive universal information/F from the environment in the form of light, sound, food, heat, cold, and/or scent. This universal information/F is adapted by the innate law, coded, transmitted through the afferent nerve of the special sense organ to a specific area of the physical brain to be decoded by the innate law for adaptation to the environment when interpreted through our educated brain.

A special sense cycle can also be made abnormal by impingement on efferent functional nerves by vertebral subluxation which would affect directly the tissue cell of the special sense organ because of interference in transmission of innate impulse.

For example, one of the nerves supplying innate impulses to the eye is the zygomatic nerve which "exits the brain stem at the pons and travels through the internal auditory canal to reach the facial canal of the temporal bone".[27] It then subdivides into several branches carrying innate impulses from the brain to many areas, one of which is the orbicularis oculi muscle responsible for closing the eyelids, protecting the eye from irritants (dust, dirt), too much light, and keeping the eye lubricated. Exiting the pons of the brain stem, it can be interfered with by vertebral subluxation. The cycle can also be made abnormal by an imbalance of body chemistry (serous circulation) resulting in abnormal metabolism of the sense organ due to vertebral subluxations anywhere in the spine.

ART. 128. HOW TO APPLY THE ABNORMAL CYCLE OF IN-COORDINATION OF ACTIVITIES

Abnormal cycles of in-coordination of activities have been demonstrated in Fig. 20 showing the concussion causing a vertebral subluxation at the vertemere (shaded boxes). Abnormal cycles are caused by interference with the transmission of the constructive innate impulse that have reverted into a deconstructive nerve impulse, which is simply a non-adapted universal information/F (Prin. 26). It also shows the modification of innate impulses conducted to the vertemere to produce a vertebral adjustment. This is the area of concern for the chiropractor in introducing the adjustic thrust in order to practice the chiropractic objective.

---

27. Zygomatic Nerve. https://anatomy.co.uk/zygomatic-nerve/ (1999-2023). June 2024

ART. 129. THE COMPLETE IN-COORDINATION OF ACTIVITIES CYCLE

This is a complex cycle combining the abnormal vertemere cycle. It involves a multitude of various compensating cycles within the body. The compensating cycles are the functional cycles of adaptation to various body parts to compensate if it is possible according to universal laws (Prin. 24) by the work of other organs or systems. Thus, if the liver fails to secrete the proper amounts of enzymes, the pancreas and other organs of intestinal digestion, under the innate control may, sometimes, compensate for the lack of work that the liver leaves undone, if it is possible, and that, not until the transmission of innate impulse is restored through the correction of vertebral subluxations.

When instantaneous integral adaptation of sensation feedback occurs under the innate control, and vertebral subluxation is detected and located, the compensating cycles are constructed through innate compensation processing (Fig. 18). Along with modifying innate impulses to correct the vertebral subluxation, various modified information/F will be constructed and conducted to different systems and organs compensating for the lack of coordination of activities manifested. This requires time (Prin. 6) for all the compensating and adaptive provisions to be established, and when that takes place, a state of synchronized frequencies of information/F exists. Prior to synchronization, it was randomized. When the vertebral adjustment is processed by the innate law the restoration of transmission of innate impulses for coordination of activities begins and compensation cycles come to a stop (Fig. 20).

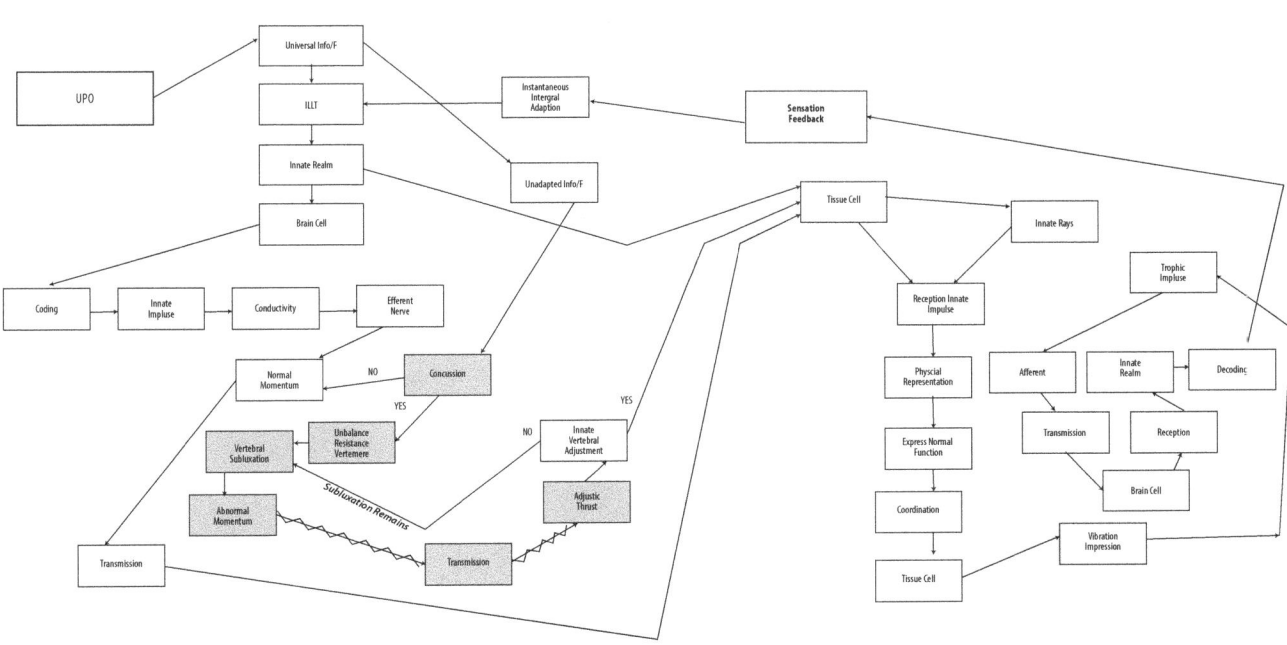

Fig. 20. Shows in this flowchart that the dark boxes as the subluxated cycle causing interference in transmission of innate impulses for coordination of activities of the vertemere that is compounded with the normal complete cycle for coordination of activities. It also shows the introduction of the adjustic thrust with the further intent that the external educated information/F it contains will be adapted by the innate law to process a vertebral adjustment. This flowchart works along all previous and subsequent flowcharts, including myriad other flowcharts, under the innate control, simultaneously.

The student is reminded that it is the lack of ease (DIS-EASE) of the neurons-transmitters comprised within the vertemere that will alter the momentum in transmission of the innate impulses. Those neurons will not transmit in a timely manner. The neuron-transmitters are not manifesting their roles and purposes violating principle 32. This is the tragic consequence of the vertebral subluxation. It is the fact that it causes incoordination of DIS-EASE from the site of the impinged neuron-transmitters at the vertemere level. However, the in-coordination of activities is throughout the whole body. The innate processing involves multiple complexities of cycles simultaneously and includes the vertemere cycle.

ART. 130. "CONDITION" AND "LOCAL"

Condition is the term used to indicate the vitality of living E/matter in the whole body, whether coordinated or uncoordinated in activities. Vitality is the soundness or integrity of tissue cells. It is the quality of liveliness of tissue cells. It is an important factor in understanding the tragic consequence of the vertebral subluxation.

This understanding includes the "condition" and "local." "Condition" pertains to the soundness of living E/matter that comes from innate rays/waves of the specifically programmed applications of the innate law to control the components of the tissue cell (cellular innate control). It is always compounded with innate impulses for coordination of activities according to universal laws (Prin. 23, 24) causing specific motions of the cell that includes the circulation of body chemistry. "Local" refers to the transmitting neurons. If these neuron-transmitters are deprived of their innate-normal complement of innate impulses due to the impingement of those neurons from the vertebral subluxation (Prin. 31), their ability to transmit with innate-normal momentum and to adapt fully is lacking ease. These neuron-transmitters are in a state of DIS-EASE (Prin. 30). When interference with transmission occurs (Prin. 29) violating the principle of coordination (Prin. 32), it causes in-coordination of activities within the whole body. The lack of ease (DIS-EASE), or the state of ease that is affecting the neuron ("local"), is an absolute due to the fact that a person has either a vertebral subluxation or does not have a vertebral subluxation which impinges the nerve that is interfering with the transmission of innate impulses. The momentum in transmission of innate impulses is either innate-normal or it is not. Since there are different locations and myo-vectors of vertebral subluxations, the in-coordination of activities of the parts of the body will manifest in different degrees.

Coordination of actions involves every tissue cell of all the parts of the body so that they have coherent actions in fulfilling their roles and purposes (Prin. 32). All the parts of the body act through interoperability and belong to an interrelated, independent organism that is affected by all of them. Every single part of the body is interconnected and adapted, under the innate control, for coordination of actions for mutual benefit (Prin. 23).

ART. 131. RESISTANCE

Resistance is the term used to indicate the ability of a tissue cell to withstand adverse environmental conditions. It is an attribute of the tissue cell's vitality and immunity, so to speak. It depends upon the constant innate control (Prin. 21). It is an aspect of the soundness of the tissue cell. It is the perfection of its structure within its limitations that is actually the tissue cell's soundness (Prin. 5, 24). The soundness of structure depends upon successful adaptation of universal information/F and E/matter by the innate law (Prin. 23) *(See Art. 133)*. Resistance counteracts the onset of deconstructive survival values, adverse conditions or very stressful environmental conditions, the rapid breeding of germs or viruses, contagion, infection, or mental and physical shocks, wherein adaptability is impaired. These are factors that determine the resistance of the body as they interact with the limitations of E/matter. The resistance of the tissue cell is dependent upon innate-normal transmission of innate impulses for coordination of activities of all the parts of the body, the innate-normal radiation/oscillation of innate rays/waves for metabolism of the body parts, and the quality of food, air, water, and many other external factors. Chiropractors address only the vertebral subluxation by practicing the chiropractic objective derived from the 33 principles of chiropractic basic's science.

REVIEW QUESTIONS FOR ARTICLES 122 - 131

1. What is the cause of incoordination of DIS-EASE?
2. What is the physical representation of the cause of DIS-EASE?
3. What is lacking ease and leads to incoordination of DIS-EASE?
4. If a body part is uncoordinated, which principle is violated?
5. What are equivalent vibrations?
6. What are equivalent impressions?
7. What are equivalent sensations?
8. What are trophic impulses/signals?
9. What is the distinction between "condition" and "local"?
10. What factors determine the resistance of the body?

ART. 132. UNSOUNDNESS

Unsoundness is the term used in chiropractic to denote a shortcoming, a lack of vitality or of wholeness of any tissue in the body. If it concerns body tissues it is called physical unsoundness. If it concerns brain/field tissue, it is computation unsoundness.

Unsoundness is a debilitation of living tissue, which of course weakens its resistance rendering it unable to counteract adverse external or internal information/F. There is also improper computation, which is an unsound brain/field activity, which concerns the activity of the educated brain, called educated control *(See Art. 53)*. Chiropractic does not concern itself with any kind of unsoundness of tissue cell. Chiropractic is concerned only with the restoration in transmission of innate impulses for coordination of activities through the location, analysis, and facilitation of the correction of vertebral subluxations.

The next section addresses a human physiology from the viewpoint of chiropractic to emphasize the interoperability of relationships between input (adapted universal information/F by the innate law), computation (innate integral processing of characterization), transmission (neuronal conduction of innate information/F), and output (cellular expression of innate information/F)*(See Vol. 1, Fig. 7)*. It underscores the importance of the correction of vertebral subluxation for the innate-normal transmission of innate impulses, which is the chiropractic objective.

ART. 133. SURVIVAL VALUES

Survival value is the term used to describe the unit of adaptation after the expression from the tissue cell of a unit of innate information/F. Survival value is the unit element of an evolutionary benefit of the organism in terms of adaptability in fulfilling its roles and purposes.

A survival value is that positive value due to an organism having adapted to its external and internal environments. Every encounter of the tissue cell with the environment is a survival value and contributes to the positive welfare of the whole body.

ART. 134. ACCUMULATIVE CONSTRUCTIVE AND DECONSTRUCTIVE SURVIVAL VALUE

The accumulating survival value can be constructive or deconstructive toward structural E/matter in accordance to the limitation of E/matter (Prin. 24). Constructive survival value is part of the vitality and soundness of the organism expressing the instructive innate information/F through motion (Prin. 13, 14). Deconstructive survival value demonstrates a lack of adaptability of the organism and will increase the limitations of E/matter and will thereby decrease the resistance of the whole body. This scenario is a prime condition for a concussion of information/F to occur causing a vertebral subluxation producing a lack of ease of the neuron-transmitters altering the momentum of the transmission of innate impulse (Prin. 29, 30, 31a). This in turn violates the principle of coordination (Prin. 32).

Dr. Claude Lessard

ART. 135. MOMENTUM

Momentum, by definition, is the product of the mass and velocity of an object. The higher the momentum, the more force will be required to stop an object. Impulse is defined as the force applied over a certain interval of time. The impulse-momentum theorem states that impulse is the change in momentum.[28]

Momentum, in chiropractic, is the motion of the transmission of the innate impulse by the nerve conductor for coordination of activities. The innate impulse is organized innate information/F into instructions for coordination of activities. The innate impulse is both immaterial (innate) and material (impulse). Information/F is the link between the non-discrete organizing principle and the discrete E/matter (Prin. 10). Therefore, the nerve conductor transmitting the innate impulse that carries the instructive message has an innate-normal momentum (Prin. 27) that can be interfered by a vertebral subluxation (Prin. 28, 29, 31a). Chiropractic never addresses the effect of vertebral subluxation regarding the expression of innate information/F by E/matter (Prin. 13). Chiropractic is concerned exclusively with the location, analysis and facilitation of the correction of vertebral subluxation, thus restoring to innate-normal the momentum in transmission of the innate impulse, nothing more, nothing less, nothing else.

ART. 136. MOMENTUM AND TIMING REGARDING INCOORDINATION OF ACTIVITIES

Momentum-[29]

    1. an inpelling force or strength

    (impulse, forcefulness, strength, force- physical energy or intensity)

    2. the product of a body's mass and its velocity

    (physical property- any property used to characterize matter and energy and their interactions)

Angular Momentum-

    1. the product of the momentum of a rotating body and its distance from the axis of rotation

Momentum is mass of E/matter multiplied by its velocity (momentum = mass x velocity). Since all processes require time and space (Prin. 6), an unbalanced momentum in transmission will always either speed up the innate impulses (> frequencies) or slow them down (< frequencies). There will be a change in velocity in time and the timing of the transmission of innate impulse will be off. The cause of the altered momentum in transmission of innate impulses is the lack of ease of the transmitting neurons caused by the vertebral subluxation (Prin. 31a). Note that the interference in momentum of transmission occurs also at the rotation level (spinning) of the innate impulses due to the angular momentum of the neuron transmitters controlled by the inforuns. The innate impulse will revert back to an un-adapted nerve impulse and will be out of sync. Thus, the instructive message will be compromised and will be expressed as such by the receptor body part causing in-coordination of activities within the whole body.

---

28. "Impulse and Momentum" The Physics Hypertextbook. physics.info/momentum/summary.shtml (1998-2024). June 2024

29. "Momentum." WordNet. wordnetweb.princeton.edu June 2024

The following diagram uses a ticker tape as an example of momentum of transmission of innate impulses out of innate normal timing:

. . . .**vs**..

Fig. 21. Demonstrates that at approximately the tenth dot on the diagram, a vertebral subluxation occurs (Prin. 31a). It causes a lack of ease of the transmitting neurons (Prin. 30). It changes the momentum of the transmission of innate impulses (Prin. 29). The crucial timing of the transmitted message carried by the innate impulse has been interfered with and now violates the principle of coordination (Prin. 32).

ART. 137. MOMENTUM AND TIMING REGARDING COORDINATION OF ACTIVITIES

When a vertebral adjustment is processed by the innate law (Prin. 31b), the momentum of the innate impulse is restored and reverts back to innate-normal (Prin. 27).

The following diagram uses a ticker tape as an example of momentum of transmission of innate impulses restored to innate normal timing:

. . . .**vs**..................**va** . . . .

Fig. 22. Demonstrates that at approximately the tenth dot on the diagram, a vertebral subluxation (vs) occurs (Prin. 31a). On the thirtieth dot the vertebral adjustment (va) is processed by the innate law correcting the vertebral subluxation (Prin. 31b). It removes the interference with the transmission of innate impulses (Prin. 29), which normalizes the momentum of the innate impulses. It restores ease of the transmitting neurons according to universal laws (Prin. 24, 31b). Thus, the crucial timing of the transmitted message carried by the innate impulse is restored to innate-normal (Prin. 6, 27) and now satisfies the principle of coordination (Prin. 32).

The next section of articles will highlight the chemistry involved in cell metabolism. It is the chemistry contained within the serums that circulate throughout the body, through the serous circulation to convey the nutrients necessary for the cell's soundness and vitality. Some cellular manifestations, which are effects, will be studied for the sole and limited purpose to demonstrate the absolute necessity for an innate-normal transmission of innate impulses, which is the aim of the chiropractic objective. We must always remember that chiropractic is exclusively about correcting the cause of the interference in transmission, which is the vertebral subluxation (Prin. 31a). Once the chiropractor introduces the adjustic thrust that has been determined by pre-checks and verified by post-checks, the cause of the interference in transmission, which is the vertebral subluxation, is now corrected (Prin. 31b). The work of the chiropractor is completed until the next spinal check since it is congruent with the chiropractic objective.

ART. 138. DEPLETION

Depletion is the manifestation of the shrinking of a cell that deviates from its innate-normal size. It is a lack of soundness of the cell. It has the capability to be repleted, if it is possible within the limitation of its E/matter (Prin. 24). The functions involved are: nutritive, reparatory, and indirectly from other body parts that produce the chemistry necessary for the metabolism of the cell (bile, enzymes, amino acids, etc.) coursing through the body serums within the serous circulation.

The student is referred to the chiropractic theory of cell expansion *(See Art. 70)*. When a cell expands and grows to its innate-normal size, the cell has reached its mature size and texture. When a depleted tissue cell within the body participates in coordination of actions on behalf of the organism, the depletion manifests within the cell's motion. It is no longer sound, it will not function normally, and it will expend contents during its attempt at secretion and excretion. If that tissue cell can be adapted by the innate law, it sometimes can recuperate and be replenished without affecting its size and construction, if it is possible according to universal laws (Prin. 24). If a tissue cell of a body part is underused, as in muscle cell, it will be depleted. However, since chiropractic is not about effects, our study is mainly to demonstrate the absolute necessity of the body to continually receive an innate-normal transmission of innate impulses for coordination of activities of all body parts. When chiropractors practice the chiropractic objective exclusively, they are always addressing the cause and not the effects.

ART. 139. DIMINUTION

Diminution of a cell is synonymous with depletion and is due to a lack of proper nutrition or a lack of coordinated functioning of some body parts. According to its chiropractic meaning the tissue cell can be replenished and does not refer to deconstruction of tissues.

ART. 140. REPLETION

Repletion is the restoration of a tissue cell to innate-normal size and soundness, when it has been depleted and it is not beyond its limitation of E/matter. It is not the same as expansion, with which the innate law originally adapted the cell. It is the reparation, in the nutritional sense of the chemistry necessary that circulates through the body's serums for replenishment and reparation, leading to innate-normal metabolism of the cell. Repletion is the return to innate-normal of a cell that has been depleted. A vertebral subluxation causes an interference with the momentum of the transmission of innate impulses for coordination of activities of the parts of the body that are involved in producing the correct balance of body chemistry for innate-normal metabolism of the cell. Therefore, for the cell to be repleted, the whole body requires adequate balanced body chemistry circulating through its serums, an innate-normal transmission of innate impulses and coordinated activities of all its parts. Chiropractic addresses the interference in transmission of innate impulses through the practice of its objective exclusively.

ART. 141. DEGENERATION

Degeneration is the deconstruction of cells, due to deterioration, that exceeded the limitation of E/matter. Degenerated tissue cannot be restored by repletion. It may have one of more signs of life, but the cell has exceeded the limitation of E/matter. It is beyond return to innate-normal function, and in the course of time the cell will die.

Since it is the innate law that adapts information/F and E/matter for use in the body, so that all parts all parts of the body will have coordinated action for mutual benefit (Prin. 23), it underscores the absolute necessity of the body to continually receive an innate-normal transmission of innate impulses.

Dr. Claude Lessard

REVIEW QUESTIONS FOR ARTICLES 132 - 141

1. What is the definition of unsoundness in chiropractic?
2. What are survival values?
3. What is the distinction between accumulative constructive and accumulative deconstructive survival values?
4. What is momentum as used in chiropractic?
5. What is depletion of tissue?
6. What is diminution of tissue?
7. What is repletion of tissue?
8. What is degeneration of tissue?
9. Differentiate between degeneration and diminution, as used in chiropractic.

ART. 142. THE CARRYING CAPABILITY OF NERVES

The function of nerve tissue is to transmit innate information/F from brain cell to tissue cell and from tissue cell to brain cell *(See Art. 62)*. Nerve tissue is used as a conductor of innate information/F. It being material, has limitations, therefore interference in transmission is possible (Prin. 5, 24, 29).

Whatever we construct with our educated intelligence exists as a principle that can be copied, as it possesses the property of copy-ability. Since we cannot give what we do not have, let us use the law of continuous supply and computation (Prin. 33) with some analogies and a comparison.

Sitting on a dock of the bay in Ocean City, N.J. during early evening twilight, in August, an amazing spectacle occurs. As the sky darkens, many different kinds of lights and sounds can be experienced. The bay becomes enchanted with signaling lights coming from boats moving across the water; with music from the shore's bars; with the green beacon from the small airport that flashes on and off. All these systems have something in common. The boats' lights, the music and the airport beacon, they are all signals. They are carrying information that can be coded, decoded and copied. These shared properties can link entities together. Boats' lights link boaters to avoid collisions with each other; the music links musician and audience bringing a delightful mood; the airport beacon links airplanes for traffic control. The fact that they can code, decode, and copy messages to connect entities is extremely important to understand existence and life. Information/F is the link that connects the non-material with the material (Prin. 10). It is at the heart of everything. The innate impulse is also capable of carrying a coded message through the conductivity of the nerve system to transmit it to a receptor body part to be decoded and acted upon because the innate law adapts information/F and E/matter for use in the body (Prin. 23).

The chiropractic objective is not attempting to improve the organizing principle that is 100% perfect. It is not attempting to improve E/matter per se, since we do not know how it should be. It is attempting to remove interference at the vertebral level that will restore transmission of conducted information/F. It aims to restore the momentum of the innate impulse because timing is most important for all activities. For example, to perform a symphony, to bake a cake, to teach a course, to play hockey, all of these activities require proper timing in order to be most effective. The activities of the human body are also subject to the momentum of coded innate impulses, for better or for worse.

Interference in transmission.

In the data communication system of the body, innate impulses go through or over the nerve system as the transmission medium (Prin. 28). This transmission medium is material and is therefore limited (Prin. 24). It literally means that the innate impulses flowing through or over the nerve system as transmission medium can be subjected to interference due to vertebral subluxations (Prin. 28, 29, 31a). This interference causes a lack of ease (DIS-EASE) of the transmitting neurons, which disturbs the momentum of transmission of the innate impulse.

The frequencies of innate impulses that are transmitted at the beginning in the brain cell are not the same as the innate impulses that are received at the end in the tissue cell. What is originally sent is not what is received. These interferences corrupt the quality of the message through untimely momentum.

There are two possible consequences:

Instructive bit errors may occur due to a change in frequencies.

Interferences may degrade the quality of the instructions that are received in an untimely manner.

Dr. Claude Lessard

Causes of interference in transmission of innate information/F:

Vertebral subluxation causing disturbance of momentum in transmission. From chiropractic's basic science, vertebral subluxations are always involved in the cause of interference in transmission whether directly or indirectly (Prin. 31a) even when trauma is the cause of the interference.

Trauma causing a distortion, that is made up of different frequencies are composite signals, due to damage of transmitting neurons.

Chiropractic is exclusively concerned with vertebral subluxation and not trauma.

Vertebral subluxation is causing disturbance in transmission. Disturbance is a change of momentum of the innate impulse that is transmitted through the nerve. When an innate impulse is transmitted through a nerve, it is propelled by the motion of the neuron-transmitters, so that it can overcome the resistance of the nerve itself as a whole. It is due to the property of elasticity of the nerve conductor. A nerve has the ability to be stretched and to be slackened. That is why a wire carrying electrical signals gets warm, if not hot, after a while. Some of the electrical energy is converted to heat in the signal. The same occurs at the site of the vertebral subluxation. The heat is a manifestation of the working muscles used by the innate law to correct the vertebral subluxation. Working muscles are the basis for identifying the vectors involved for ADIO analysis. This heat is also an indicator to determine when and when not to perform the adjustic thrust for the neurocalograph pattern analysis. With the electrical wire, engineers use amplifiers to amplify the signals to compensate for this loss. In chiropractic, chiropractors locate, analyze the vertebral subluxation and they introduce a specific adjustic thrust for a vertebral adjustment to be processed by the innate law (Prin. 31b). This figure shows the effect of attenuation and amplification:

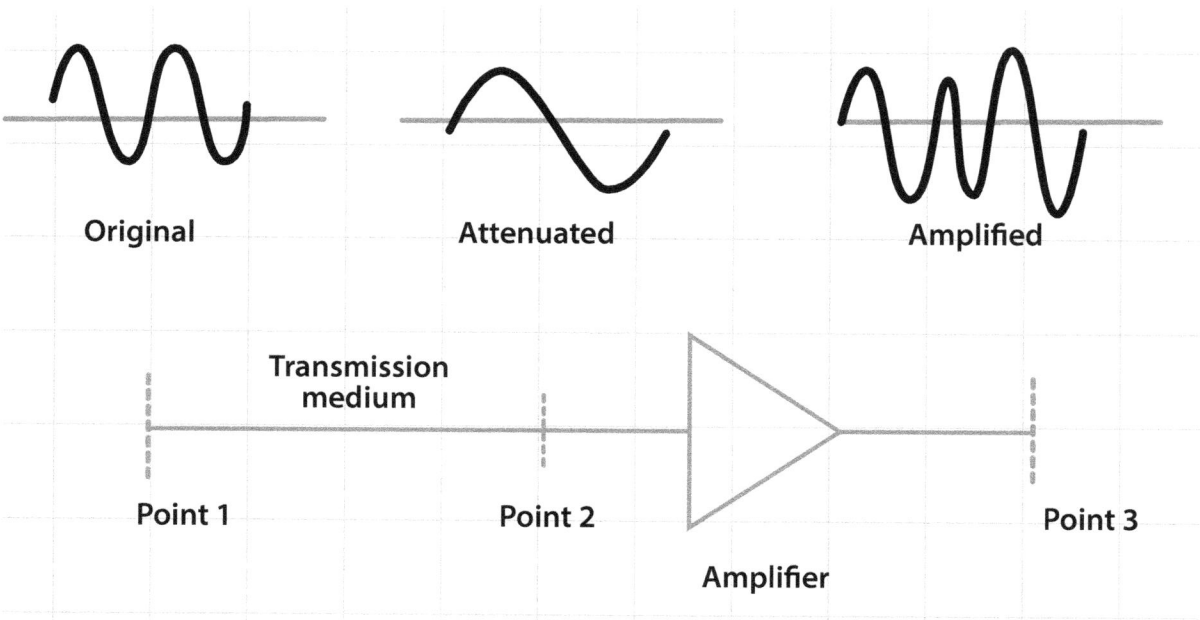

Fig. 23a. Demonstrates interference in electromagnetic signal impulse transmission and its compensation through amplification. When signal has lost or gained its strength, for this purpose engineers use the concept of decibel (dB). Decibel is used to measure the relative strengths of two signals or a signal at two different points. If a signal is attenuated then dB is negative and if a signal is amplified so the dB is positive.

Here is the figure constructed into a chiropractic diagram showing the effect of vertebral subluxation and a vertebral adjustment:

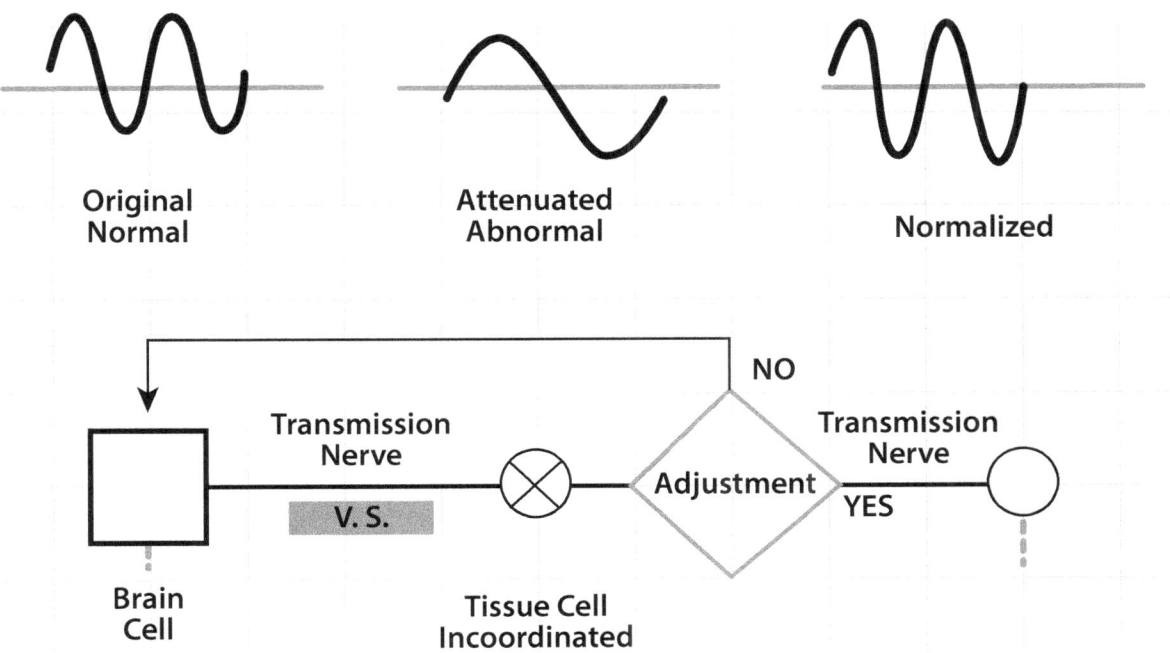

Fig. 23b. Demonstrates the vertebral subluxation and the effect it has on the disturbance (change) in momentum of the transmission of the innate impulse and its normalization through a vertebral adjustment. The innate impulse originates from the brain cell to be propelled through nerves and transmitted to a tissue cell of the body part for coordination of activities. When a subluxation occurs the momentum in transmission of the innate impulse is disturbed resulting in the in-coordination of the tissue cell of the body part. When the vertebral adjustment is processed by the innate law (Prin. 31b), the normalization in transmission is restored, if it is possible according to universal laws (Prin. 24), and the tissue cell of the body part is now coordinated. The tissue cell of the body part must also be sound in order to manifest coordination of action (Prin. 32).

Trauma causing a distortion is made up of different frequencies that are composite instructions due to damage of transmitting neurons.

Distortion

If a message changes its form or shape, it is referred to as distortion. It is corrupted data. Information/F of that kind is made up of different frequencies that are composite signal impulses un-adapted and reverted to universal information/F, which are deconstructive toward structural E/matter (Prin. 26). Distortion occurs in these composite signal impulses. Each component of frequency has its propagation speed traveling through a medium. Therefore, different components have different delays in arriving at the final destination (Prin. 6). These composite information/F have different phases at the receiver than they did at the source.

This figure shows the effect of distortion on a composite signal impulse:

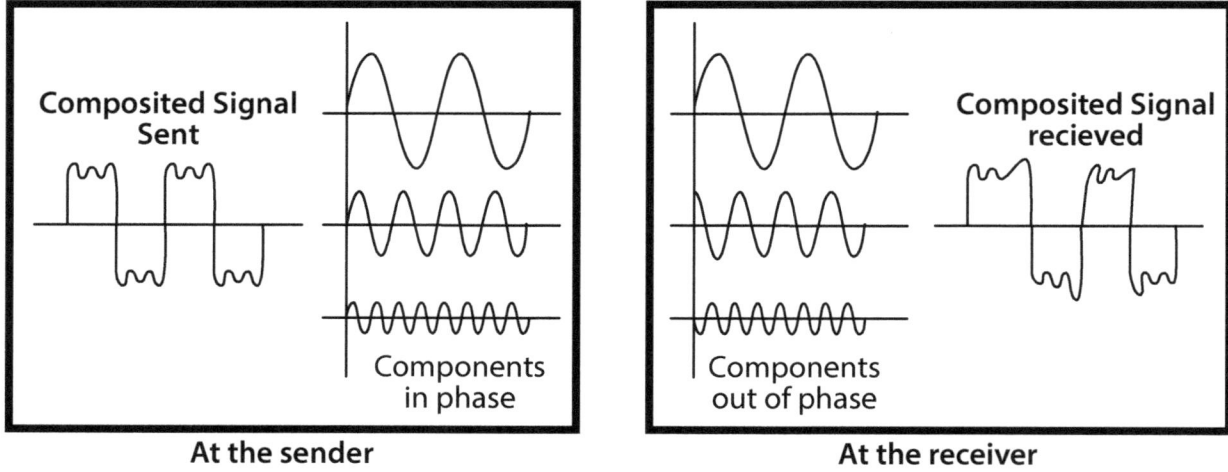

Fig. 24. Demonstrates trauma and its composite effect on the transmitted distortion for comparative purpose only. Chiropractic does not address trauma.

Once again, the student is reminded that chiropractic is exclusively concerned with vertebral subluxation and not trauma. This comparative study is to differentiate the consequences of both interferences. Inasmuch as trauma is a possible cause of interference in transmission, chiropractors exclusively locate, analyze and facilitate the correction of vertebral subluxations.

ART. 143. THE RESTORATION CYCLE FOR COORDINATION OF ACTIVITIES

The restoration cycle is a complex cycle consisting of the abnormal, compensation, normal and vertemere cycles for coordination of activities. It is how abnormal is restored to innate-normal in the vertemere cycle, through the correction of vertebral subluxations to remove the compensation cycle for coordination of activities. Follow the steps of the flow chart in Fig. 20, starting with the unbalanced resistance at the vertemere for cycle clarification.

ART. 144. THE PRACTICAL CYCLE FOR COORDINATION OF ACTIVIVITES

This practical cycle for coordination of activities is paramount to the practice of chiropractic. It is a complex cycle consisting of all the steps of the normal complete cycle for coordination of activities, the abnormal cycle, the vertemere cycle and the restoration cycle. *(See Fig. 20)*. It is indicative of how chiropractic does WHAT it does and WHY. It reveals that chiropractic does not add anything to the body nor does it take away anything from the body either. Chiropractic restores the transmission of innate impulses so they can be normalized, from within, by the innate law through the practice of its objective.

ART. 145. THE SEROUS CIRCULATION AS A MAJOR INSTRUMENT OF COORDINATION BY THE INNATE LAW

The ability of a tissue cell of a body part to coordinate depends upon its soundness and vitality as well as the timely innate impulses it receives (Prin. 5). The tissue cell of the body part must not only have 100%/perfect innate impulses in order to function properly; it must also have 100%/perfect soundness and vitality of structure in order to decode these innate impulses properly.

Since the tissue cells of the body part obtain their biochemical nutrients via the circulation of body chemistry, it is necessary that the serous circulation be innate-normal, in order that the cells of the body parts coordinate perfectly.

The serous circulation is a chiropractic concept that connects the theory of information/F of the body function and the theory of body chemistry, both of which are vitalistic in their approach. Consequently, the serous circulation is itself vitalistic.

The serous circulation is directly under the innate control. It is the function of the innate law to adapt information/F and E/matter for use in the body so that all parts of the body will have coordination of action for mutual benefit (Prin. 23). Therefore, the soundness and vitality of all the tissue cells of the body and the timely reception of their innate impulses are absolutely necessary for coordination of activities. It underscores the necessity for the innate-normal transmission of innate impulses. Chiropractic addresses exclusively the timely transmission of innate impulses through the practice of its objective.

ART. 146. THE SEROUS CIRCULATION OF BODY CHEMISTRY

The serous circulation is the course of water through the body of an organism carrying body chemistry and nutrients to all the cells, and carrying away from them their used products. It is done primarily via blood and lymph to facilitate the transportation chemistry, nutrients, and oxygen to all the cells of the body, in addition to removing the waste product from all the cells of the body in order to maintain an efficient metabolism of all the cells of the body.

The tissue cell's ability to sense through specialized applications and process fluctuation of internal chemistry levels is a requisite for the soundness of the cell. Chemistry and nutrients continually course through the serous system in order to be selected through cellular processes. The innate law uses specific component parts, as sensors, of the circulation of body chemistry to track down intracellular and extracellular level of particulates, such as, metabolites, proteins, lipids, sugars, amino acids, to integrate and coordinate the metabolism of all the tissue cells of the body employing hormones to provide soundness and vitality to the cells.

Body chemistry and nutrients are substances (adapted and computed by the innate law) involved in biochemical reactions composed of cellular material that circulate through the waters of the serous circulation. These waters convey food, oxygen, and other chemical elements to all the cells of the body. Once the cellular intake process is completed, the waters of the serous circulation remove heat, carbon dioxide and other chemicals that are waste products of cellular metabolism. This circulation of the waters from the environment through the body and back again to the environment is the serous cycle for soundness and vitality of all the cells of the body. The circulation of body chemistry requires coordination of activities of all the parts of the body to benefit the whole. Thus, it is necessary for all the body parts to have innate-normal transmission of innate impulses in order to convey the innate-normal cellular nutritional balance and the carrying out of innate-normal cellular waste products through the serous circulation. Here are three diagrams illustrating some components of the serous circulation of body chemistry:

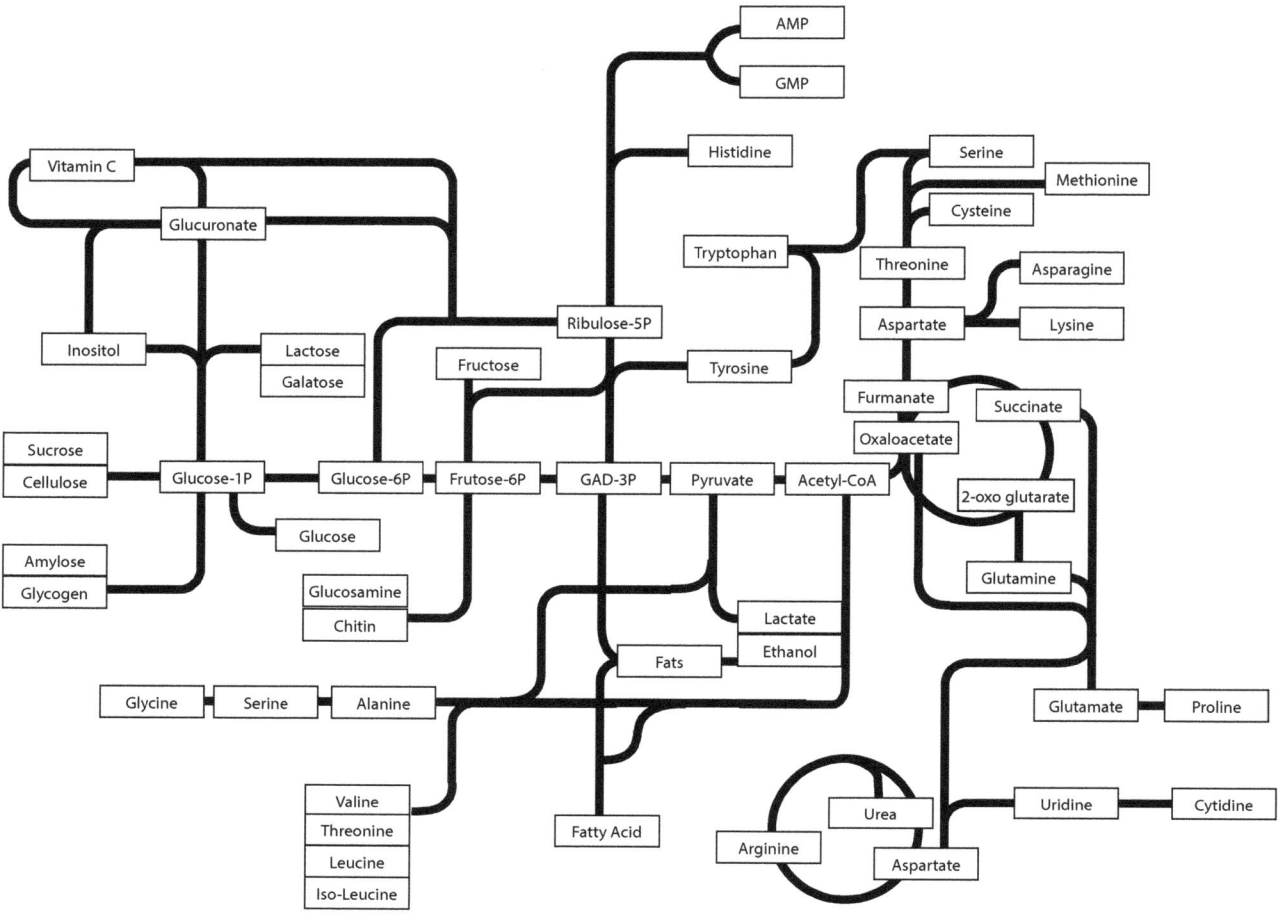

Fig. 25. Illustrates the circulation of some nutrients necessary of cellular metabolism.

The 2027 Chiropractic Textbook Volume 2

BODY CHEMISTRY CIRCULATION

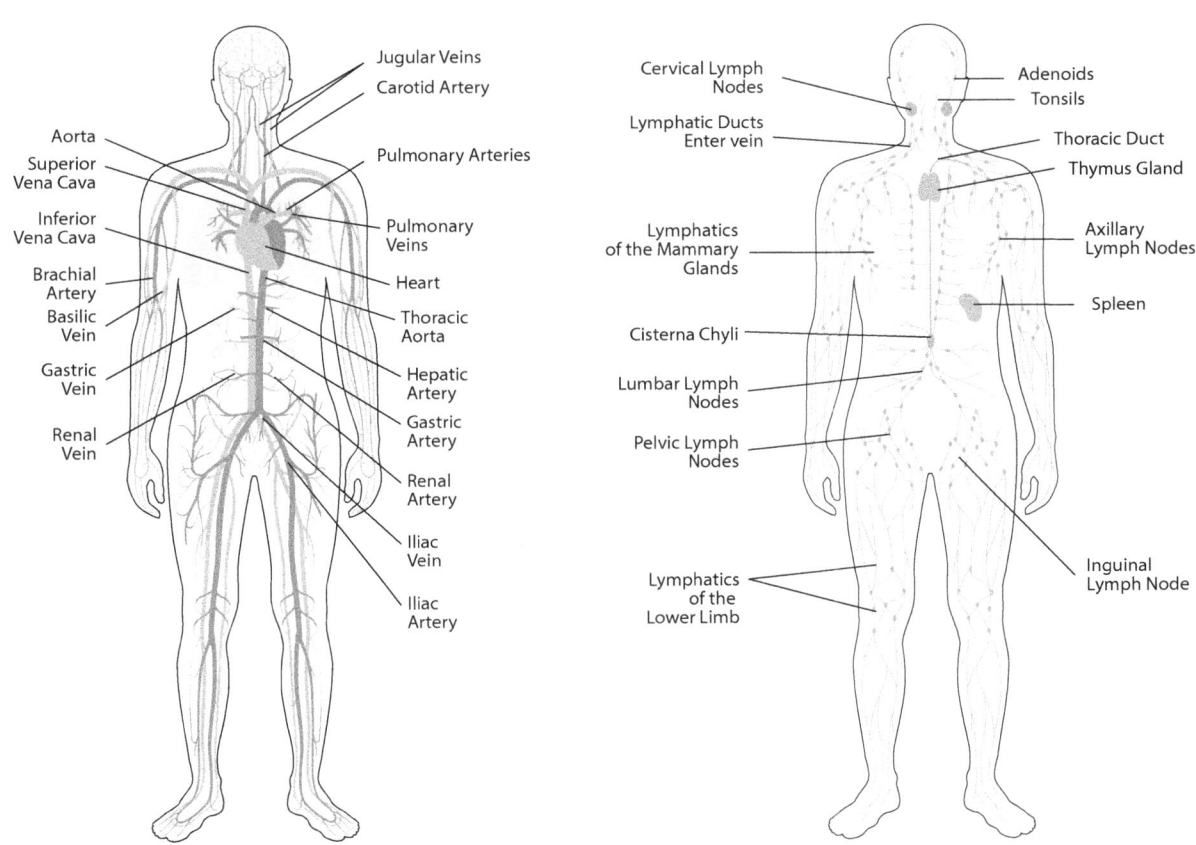

Fig. 26. Two diagrams illustrating the circulation of body chemistry: First, (a) through blood conveying nutrients and oxygen to the cells and carrying away carbon dioxide from the cells, and second (b), through lymph removing cellular waste materials.

The percentage of water in the body is around 65%; the rest is solid E/matter that is comprised of mostly protides. Protides, according to the dictionary are any of a class of compounds comprising the proteins and their hydrolysis products (as amino acids, amines, and amides). This percentage is maintained by the innate law as a constant innate-normal balance of input and output of water regardless of excess intake or lack of it, according to universal laws (Prin. 24, 27). This sustained balance is required by the parameters of the tissue cells that are depending upon the coordination of activities of the parts of the body. It reveals the necessity for the innate-normal transmission of innate impulses to all the body parts.

ART. 147. A CONTEMPORARY ANALOGY

For comparison let us use a pancake, which is composed of dusty particles (electrons, protons and neutrons) of flour and water. In order to have the pancake of the proper consistency it must contain the right amount of water, mixed with the flour. Any more than the required amount of water will make a pancake too wet and any less will make it too dry or lumpy. If inadequately mixed, this pancake might be too wet or too lumpy in spots.

A person is also composed of dusty particles of biological E/matter and water. The amount of water for a person's body is about 65%. More than 75% makes the body too wet in consistency, and less than 50% makes it too dry or lumpy; a person's body may be too wet or too dry in spots. To have the right balance of water circulating through the serous system, a body must have an innate-normal transmission of innate impulses for coordination of activities of all the parts of the body.

ART. 148. CONDITION OF VITALITY

Condition of vitality is the soundness of a tissue cell. Vitality is dependent upon the quality of liveliness of all the parts of the body, including the integrity of the body's chemistry serum. Therefore, the vertebral subluxation can indirectly affect the vitality of the cell due to the fact that the cell is dependent on the integrity of the circulation and the quality of body chemistry, which in turn is dependent on the coordinated activity of all the parts of the body *(See Fig. 25)* (Prin. 31a, 32). Interference in transmission (Prin. 29) always alters the momentum of the innate impulses and affects the coordination of activities of all the body parts including the serous circulation, which in turn affects the whole body. That's why interference with the transmission of innate information/F causes in-coordination *OF* DIS-EASE. It is the lack of ease (DIS-EASE) being at the site of the transmitting neurons, due to the vertebral subluxation, which is disturbing the momentum in transmission of innate impulses, that causes the incoordination of action of body parts. It is an in-coordination coming from DIS-EASE (lack of ease) of the neuron-transmitters (Prin. 29, 30). The wholeness of the body is dependent on the integrity of the serous circulation for its condition of vitality, which in turn, is dependent upon coordination of activities resulting from innate-normal transmission of innate impulses.

Despondent serum will not be effective in nurturing any tissue cell even when the cell is getting a normal transmission of innate impulses. This despondent serum will affect the adaptability of the tissue cells making them unsound, having less vitality. Therefore, both innate-normal transmission of innate impulses and soundness of the tissue cell are necessary for coordination of activities. The chiropractic objective is exclusively the location, analysis, and facilitation of the correction of vertebral subluxations for an innate- normal transmission of innate impulses.

ART. 149. SEGMENTS OF THE SEROUS CIRCULATION OF BODY CHEMISTRY

The three segments of the serous circulation are: efferent, peripheral, and afferent. This is a purely chiropractic concept of the flow of the circulation of body chemistry. The efferent flow conveys the plasma of the blood stream in the arteries, driven to the periphery by the heart. The peripheral segment is the course of the serum through the intercellular and intracellular spaces. The afferent segment is the return to environment through the lymph from the organs of elimination. The afferent bloodstream may also be considered a part of the afferent segment, insofar as it transports cellular waste materials to the organs of elimination.

The serous circulation is a chiropractic concept that explains a circulatory cycle from environment to periphery and back to environment. Every action of the body is dependent upon adapted information/F (innate impulses, innate rays, trophic impulses/signals, etc.) and E/matter (body chemistry). There are numerous chemicals with multiple functions that are being conveyed through the serum to provide the cell all of what its parameters require. The circulation of body chemistry is an important aspect to understand the necessity for an innate-normal transmission of innate impulses, that coordinates all of the activities of body parts that are used for the proper balance of the serum's body chemistry, conveyed through the serous circulation.

ART. 150. THE EFFERENT SEROUS STREAM OF BODY CHEMISTRY

The efferent serous stream is the plasma of the blood. It is the initial part of the circulation of body chemistry. Blood consists of plasma (90% water), proteins, ions, nutrients, leucocytes, erythrocytes, platelets and other bio-chemicals. It easily demonstrates the amazing process of the innate law as 100%/perfect biological software computing moment to moment, all of the adaptive challenges of the living body to be used for this purpose. The liquid, which is the vehicle for the blood, something to be pumped by the heart, is water, but water that contains the necessary nutritive materials for all the trillions of tissue cells. The red blood cells convey oxygen for the cells. The efferent serous stream carries to the tissue cells carbon, oxygen, minerals, enzymes, and various body chemistry processed and computed by the innate law. The entire serous circulation is a compilation of many systems in the body that demonstrates the movement of fluids transporting body chemistry and how these fluids supply nutrients to the tissue cell. They also carry unused body chemistry, and waste materials away from the tissue cell on the afferent side of the serous circulation.

ART. 151. THE PERIPHERAL SEGMENT OF THE SEROUS CIRCULATION OF BODY CHEMISTRY

The peripheral segment of the serous circulation is the flow of serum through the intercellular and intracellular spaces. The spaces around and between the cells, even those without cell walls, are called intercellular spaces. As nutrients conveyed by the serum are absorbed within the cells for metabolism, the waste materials are carried out to the organs of elimination. The spaces within the cells are called intracellular spaces.

While in the blood stream the body chemistry is called plasma and while in the tissue spaces it is called serum. The unused plasma returns by way of the veins to transport the blood afferently to be reused and to eliminate CO_2. The unused materials are carried away, mainly through the lymphatic system, to the organs of elimination for waste disposal or are recycled and reprocessed through the glands of the afferent segment of the serous circulation for reuse by other cells. All of these movements of fluids containing body chemistry are completely controlled and balanced by the innate law. It once again points to the absolute necessity to have an innate-normal transmission of innate impulses (Prin. 27), which is the chiropractic objective.

Intercellular And Intracellular Serous Circulation Of Body Chemistry

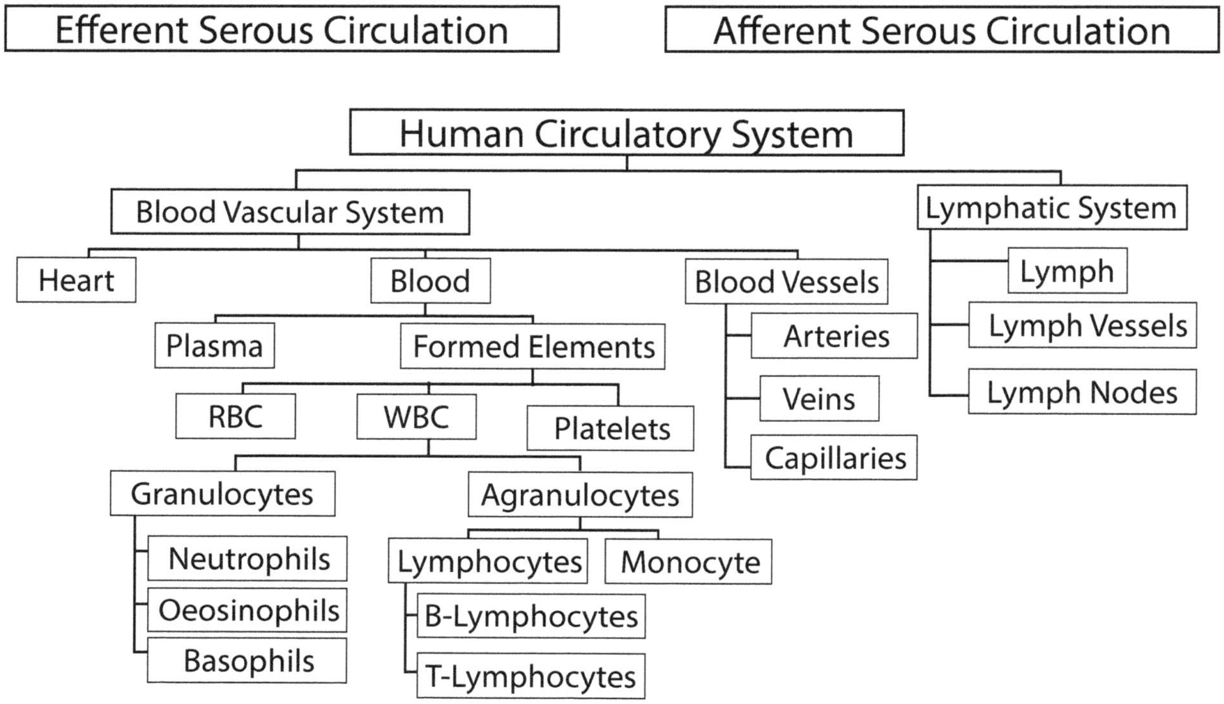

| Efferent Serous Circulation | Afferent Serous Circulation |

- **Human Circulatory System**
  - **Blood Vascular System**
    - Heart
    - Blood
      - Plasma
      - Formed Elements
        - RBC
        - WBC
          - Granulocytes
            - Neutrophils
            - Oeosinophils
            - Basophils
          - Agranulocytes
            - Lymphocytes
              - B-Lymphocytes
              - T-Lymphocytes
            - Monocyte
        - Platelets
    - Blood Vessels
      - Arteries
      - Veins
      - Capillaries
  - **Lymphatic System**
    - Lymph
    - Lymph Vessels
    - Lymph Nodes

Fig. 27a

PERIPHERAL SEROUS CIRCULATION OF BODY CHEMISTRY

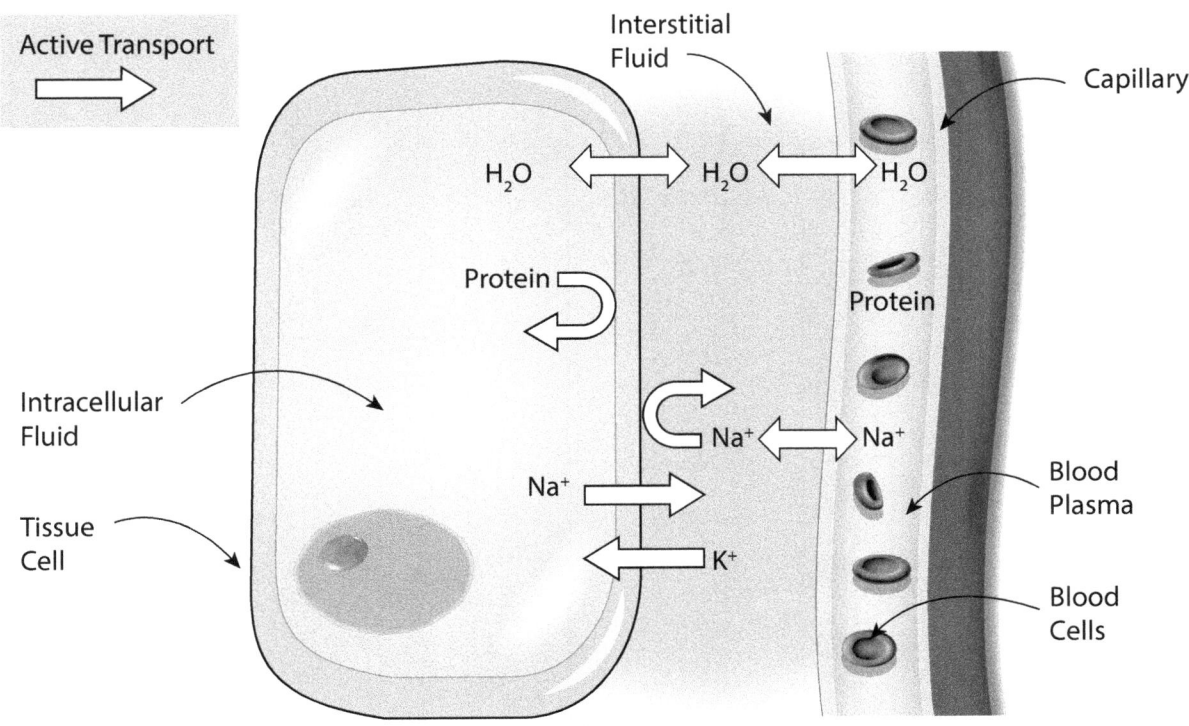

Fig. 27b.

Fig. 27a. and b. Illustrates the three segments of the serous circulation of body chemistry. The formed elements and plasma circulate through the efferent segment to the peripheral segment and away from the peripheral segment though afferent segment.

Dr. Claude Lessard

REVIEW QUESTIONS FOR ARTICLES 142 - 151

1. What tissue cells are transmitters of innate impulse in the living human body?
2. Is a vertebral subluxation the only interference with transmission of innate impulses?
3. What is the restoration cycle for coordination of activities?
4. What is the practical cycle for coordination of activities?
5. What part does the serous circulation of body chemistry play in coordination of activities?
6. What is the serous circulation of body chemistry?
7. What is the approximate percentage of water in the body?
8. How does the serous circulation of body chemistry affect the soundness of tissues?
9. Name the three segments of the serous circulation of body chemistry.
10. What is the efferent serous stream?
11. Describe the peripheral segment of the serous circulation of body chemistry.

The 2027 Chiropractic Textbook Volume 2

ART. 152. SERUM AND UREA

The serum that soaks the cell is a liquid that contains body chemistry including nutrients to be assimilated by the cell itself through a quality called applicability (app). It involves a specific cellular application for decoding information/F by the innate law within the innate field of the cell itself, according to this unique cell's parameters. It is only specific nutrients that will be assimilated by an individual cell for its metabolism. It is the process of cellular assimilation, which is a sign of life (Prin. 18). It is specific to each individual cell within the body of a living thing. It is analogous to a cell phone app that can process only specific data that is applicable exclusively to this particular app and no other.

The liquid going to the cell that is applicable to its parameters for assimilation is called serum. The cell ejects into the serous stream the material it has processed. It reveals the ability of the innate law of the cell to decode particular frequencies of information/F without interference from other frequencies that are not applicable to its specific parameters. Through this cellular application, each cell has the property of being selective under innate control. Each cell selectively takes something from the serous stream and puts something into it.

It is possible if a tissue cell is unsound that its resistance is lowered, making its ability to process materials more limited. It is then impossible to prevent invasive information/F, that causes an imbalance, without breaking a universal law (Prin. 24), which could cause a vertebral subluxation. Some unsuitable contaminants could penetrate the cell's components and possibly poison the cell due to its inability to counteract the toxins. The soundness of the tissue cell is dependent upon the quality of liveliness of all the parts of the body including the integrity of the body's serum for its metabolism *(See Art. 148)*. It underscores the importance to practice the chiropractic objective. Chiropractic is always about what is possible without breaking a universal law.

ART. 153. THE AFFERENT SEROUS STREAM

The lymph streams discharge as small channels into the larger streams. Those lymphatic vessels conduct the serous stream via an afferent pathway. Lymphatic vessels contain many nodes called lymphatic glands. Each gland processes body chemistry waste. The larger of these glands are endocrine glands, also called ductless glands, due to the fact that their chemistries are released directly into the blood circulation.

Kidney bean shaped lymphatic glands produce hormones that are transported through the vascular circulation. The serous flow infiltrates them on the convex side through the inter-cellular and intra-cellular spaces, and is adapted, processed, and controlled by the innate law to be useful for the tissue cells (Prin. 23). The serous flow leaves the glands by the concave side and is called hilum.

ART. 154. INNATE-LABORATORIES

The glands of the body are laboratories used by the innate law to process body chemistry for supply of chemicals and enzymes to the cells. These glands are controlled by the innate law to produce chemicals or substances for the use in the body, as long as they are sound, and have coordination of activities. Any substance not adapted by the innate law remains universal information/F and is deconstructive to the body (Prin. 26). It is called a poison.

The economy of data computation of the innate law, as a 100%/perfect software, continuously processes information/F and E/matter for use in the body and for coordination of activities (Prin. 23, 33). A chemical or substance, that has been assimilated by a tissue cell and is no longer usable by that particular tissue cell, may be useful to different tissue cells remarkably if those materials can be adapted and reorganized to suitable substance for other tissue cells. Therefore, no substance is eliminated if it can be of use for other cells. A classic example is a bear that hibernates will use its own inner substance to remain alive, producing very little waste as some of those waste products are adapted, computed, processed, and are used by the body of the starved animal. On the other hand, an over-fed bear during the summer will profusely eliminate this material that may contain some undigested nutrients. This excess material becomes impossible to process without breaking a universal law (Prin. 24). Chiropractic is always about what is possible. We should never underestimate the innate law, for its purpose is to maintain the body of a living thing alive (Prin. 21). This is unique for every living thing. Only limitation of E/matter can limit the innate law.

Thus, we realize again the absolute relevance of practicing the chiropractic objective in order to satisfy the principle of coordination of action (Prin. 32).

ART. 155. THE POISON POSSIBILITIES OF SERUM

Any body chemistry that is no longer usable in body metabolism and is retained in the serous circulation is a poison. Any substance, even food that is in excess for the use of the cells of the body, is a poison. Urea not being eliminated by a cell or a gland producing it is a poison to that cell or gland. Any body chemistry not adapted by the innate law or not manufactured by the cells or glands of the body is a poison. Any body chemistry in the wrong place in the body is a poison. Any non-adaptable substance in the body, be it liquid, solid, or gaseous, even if not chemically active, is a poison.

Too much water in the serum is a poison, the serum is saturated, not enough water in the serum then the serum is dehydrated. It is a poison. If the serum is abnormal, it is a poison since it cannot flow properly and soon becomes laden with urea.

There is an innate-normal amount of water that is required for the body to be maintained in balance. This number is different from person to person ranging from 45-75%; the average is about 65%. The innate law will maintain water balance for a particular body's parameters within innate-normal, which is time sensitive; otherwise compensations in the body will begin under innate control. The momentum of the transmission of innate impulses must be innate-normal for the body to have adequate water balance. It is important to exclusively practice the chiropractic objective.

ART. 156. THE END OF THE SEROUS CYCLE

Full of used materials and heat, the serum arrives at the kidneys and skin. These organs eliminate the heat and urea that are no longer usable, and excrete them from the body back to the environment. The heat and urea leave the whole body in a similar way to that in which they leave a tissue cell.

ART. 157. THE KIDNEYS

The kidneys are the organs that are the end point of the serous cycle. They have ducts leading from them, but not leading to them. The kidneys and the liver have reached maximum innate-economy when controlled by the innate law to process the urea, and has utilized all the potential of body chemistry. If the kidneys excrete usable materials, it is because those materials are not then necessary for metabolism at the moment, or have not been properly processed or manufactured for metabolism.

The excretion of the kidneys is called urine. It is manufactured for the purpose of excretion from the body. It is made from urea and of waste materials and is called elimination. It indicates the property of applicability (app) of the kidneys for the innate law to decode the information/F regarding the selectivity required for elimination. It reveals an innate-normal 100%/perfect innate law software processing information/F and E/matter for use in the body (Prin. 23, 27). The ejection of the eliminated material is called excretion, one of the signs of life (Prin. 18).

ART. 158. THE SKIN

The skin is the largest organ in the body containing many glands, which are also end points of the serous cycle. These glands eliminate urea as they eject the waste materials from the body, also actualizing part of the sign of life called excretion (Prin. 18).

ART. 159. EXCESS WATER SERUM (HYPERHYDRATION)

Excess water serum indicates the condition when there is too much water in the serum. It is called hyperhydration. It may be local or general.

When there is too much water in the serum, it fills the inter spaces and intra spaces beyond innate-normal (Prin. 27). With excess water, the serum does not flow fast enough and becomes "stagnant", that is laden with waste materials poisoning the cells. An analogy may be used to explain excess water local and general. An irrigated field may contain a balanced amount of water. The whole field may have excess water; or it may have excess water in spots. Again, it may have excess water all over, except in spots which may be have insufficient water, and vice versa.

The excretion of water in the body must always balance the intake of water and the supply of water must be adequate (average is about 65%). Thus, hyperhydration may occur in the following ways:

    1. A supply of water is constant with a lack of excretion of water.

    2. An over supply of water accompanied with a lack of excretion of water.

    3. An over supply of water accompanied with an excretion of water that is constant.

If the supply of water is innate-normal (Prin. 27), any of these factors will be adapted to coordinate or compensate for one or more that are not innate-normal, in order to keep the balance of body water constant (average 65%).

Too much water in the body adds to deconstructive survival values that the innate law must process if it is possible without breaking a universal law (Prin. 24). We see the importance of the correction of vertebral subluxations, by the innate law, to restore to innate-normal transmission the innate impulses and satisfy the principle of coordination (Prin. 31a, 31b, 32).

ART. 160. INSUFFICIENT WATER SERUM (DEHYDRATION)

Insufficient water serum indicates the condition when there is not enough water in the serum. It is called dehydration. It may be local or general.

When there is not enough water in the serum, the spaces are beneath innate-normal (Prin. 27). The serum flows too slowly and become "stagnant", that is laden with waste materials poisoning the cells. In certain areas in the body the serum may become too thick, producing friction and heat. The innate-normal flow of nutritive materials and body chemistry cannot exist for lack of proper serous circulation. Thus, dehydration may occur in the following ways:

1. A supply of water is constant with an excess of excretion of water.

2. An under supply of water accompanied with an excess of excretion of water.

3. An under supply of water accompanied with an excretion of water that is constant.

If the supply of water is innate-normal (Prin. 27), any of these factors will be adapted to coordinate or compensate for one or more that are not innate-normal, in order to keep the balance of body water constant (about 65%).

Too little water in the body adds to deconstructive survival values that the innate law must process if it is possible without breaking a universal law (Prin. 24). We see the importance of correcting vertebral subluxations, by the innate law, to restore to innate-normal transmission the innate impulses and satisfy the principle of coordination (Prin. 31a, 31b, 32).

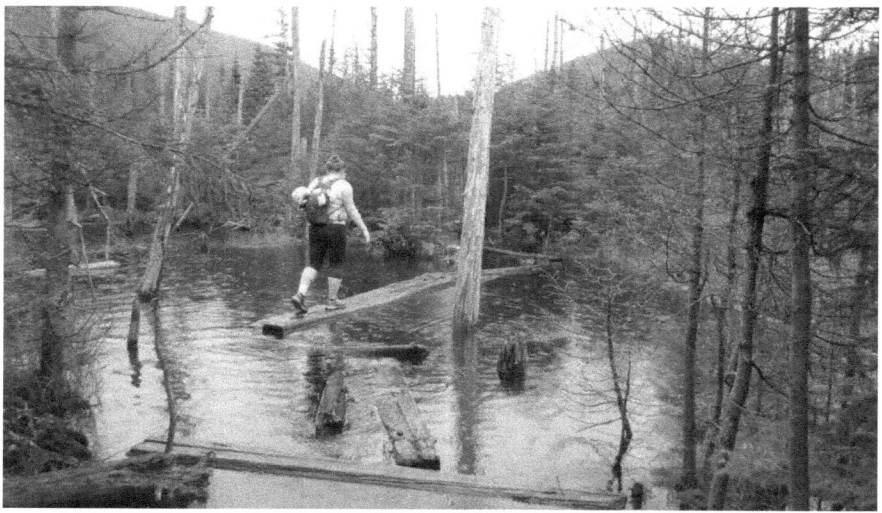

Fig. 28a *Photo Credit: Amanda Janiec*

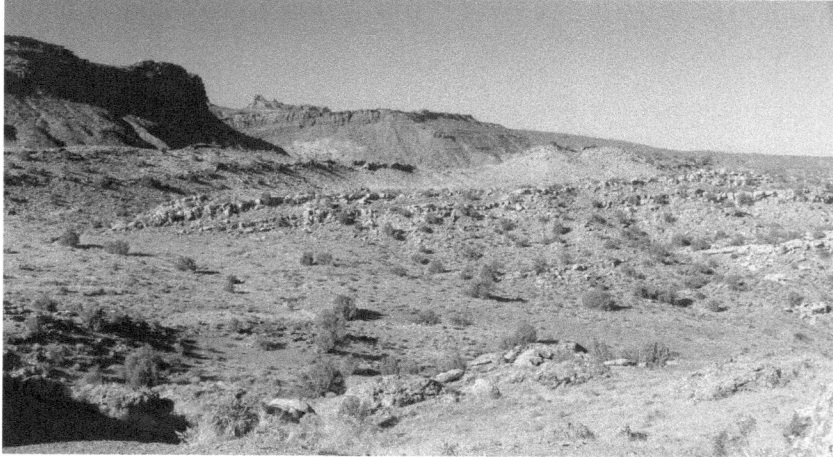

Fig. 28b *Photo Credit: Darren Williams*

Fig. 28. Excess water and insufficient water example images.

ART. 161. EFFERENT SERUM POISONING

Efferent serum poisoning occurs when the tissues are supplied with serum that is rich beyond innate-normal (Prin. 27). It is forced upon the cells on the efferent side of the serous circulation *(See Fig. 27)*. It may be local or general. It is not to be confused with edema, where the accumulation of serous fluid occurs in the tissue spaces or a body cavity without poisoning the body.

Efferent serum poisoning can be due to too much food intake. It upsets the balance of body chemistry. This really underscores the importance to properly use our educated intelligence. One should listen to the body, to choose to be moderate, and give it what it requires rather than give it a lot of everything and require the innate law sort it out. Remember that the innate law will adapt information/F and E/matter only if it is possible according to universal laws (Prin. 24).

Dr. Claude Lessard

REVIEW QUESTIONS FOR ARTICLES 152 - 161

1. What is the difference between serum and urea?
2. What is the afferent serous stream?
3. What are innate laboratories?
4. What is a poison?
5. Name the poison possibilities of serum.
6. Describe the ending of the serous cycle of body chemistry.
7. What part do the kidneys play in the serous cycle of body chemistry?
8. Differentiate between urea and urine.
9. What part does the skin play in the serous cycle of body chemistry?
10. What is meant by hyperhydration?
11. What is meant by dehydration?
12. What are the ways in which excess water serum may occur?
13. What are the ways in which insufficient water serum may occur?
14. What is efferent serum poisoning?
15. Differentiate between elimination and excretion.

ART. 162. AFFERENT SERUM POISONING

Afferent serum poisoning occurs when the urea is not removed from the cell bodies or from the immediate vicinity of the cells. Waste materials are retained at the cell and its afferent flow, which is not rapid enough, causing poor elimination and poisoning of the cells.

As an analogy, let us use grainfields of Québec. When I was a child, I noticed that the cornfield and the wheatfield of the farmer next door were separated by a dirt road. One year, corn was growing on one side while wheat was growing on the other side. The next year is it was the reverse. I asked the farmer why he was doing that. He said that it was because his father told him that it produced a better crop of both by alternating sides. Later on, I came to learn that the waste material produced by the corn was saturating the soil that was not conducive to growing corn the following year. However, if the corn was planted somewhere else it was very fruitful. The same thing happened with wheat. So, the farmer alternated the fields from both side of the road and his crops were always good, everything else being equal (water and sunshine.) What was happening was that the soil of the field was being "poisoned" by the waste material of the corn and the next season corn could not grow as well but wheat could. And the same thing happened with the wheat.

The innate-economy of data processing is always effective as long as there is no interference to the flow of its conducted innate information/F for coordination of activities. In the case of crops productivity, a simple switching of fields seems to restore its flow. In the body, the practice of the chiropractic objective is what is required to remove interference to the flow of conducted innate information/F for coordination of activities.

ART. 163. UNSOUNDNESS FROM EXCESS WATER SERUM

Unsoundness from excess water serum pertains to the lack of vitality of body tissues due to water poisoning that results from above innate-normal water serum. It could be called septic unsoundness. It is an imbalance of body chemistry. Chiropractic is only concerned with the practice of its objective.

ART. 164. UNSOUNDNESS FROM INSUFFICIENT WATER SERUM

Unsoundness from insufficient water serum pertains to the lack of vitality of body tissue due to water poisoning that results from a below innate-normal water serum. It could be called sterile unsoundness. It is an imbalance of body chemistry. Chiropractic is only concerned with the practice of its objective.

ART. 165. A CHIROPRACTIC DISCOVERY

According to Mabel Palmer, D.C., Ph.C. in her 1920 book, the serous circulation is an original theme discovered by B.J. Palmer, D.C., Ph.C. "Serous Circulation is an original theme, and my aim is to present these thoughts as briefly, yet as lucidly, as possible… We, as chiropractors, take great pride in the fact that the establishing of a serous circulation belongs to Chiropractic and is due to B. J. Palmer, who labored long and hard to prove that there is no other function so absolutely necessary to the maintenance of life as is the Serous Circulation." [30]

---

30. Palmer, Mabel H. "Anatomy." 4th ed., Davenport, IA: The Palmer School of Chiropractic- Chiropractic Fountain Head. (1920) p. 317

Dr. Claude Lessard

Chiropractic does not claim to have discovered the cycle of blood circulation, or the cycle of serum, or the cycle of lymphatic stream and its vessels and glands, as it has been known for a very long time, in the inner spaces and intra spaces of the cells. Chiropractic claims the discovery of the connection between these three great cycles, as has been explained in the previous articles. All of the body chemistry flowing through all the fluids is absolutely necessary to maintain the body alive, which is the purpose of the innate law (Prin. 21). The interoperability of innate information/F of the tissues and the organs and the glands of the body is a unique discovery of chiropractic (Prin. 20, 21, 23). The innate law is 100%/perfect and an infinite software that adapts a continuous supply of universal information/F. It assembles, computes, processes, and codes it into innate impulses utilizing the nerve system as the conductor to transmit those innate impulses for coordination of activities of the body parts (Prin. 23, 32). The innate law also governs the serous circulation utilizing arterial, venal, and lymphatic vessels to transport body chemistry for the vitality and soundness of the body parts. Innate rays/waves that emanate directly from within each cell are also involved in cellular metabolism in order to maintain the body alive. Chiropractic concerns itself exclusively with the interference of transmission-momentum of innate impulses through the location, analysis, and facilitation of the correction of vertebral subluxations.

WORLD AND LIFE VIEW POINTS

Before we address the next set of articles, it is paramount to understand there are really basically two frames of reference regarding a world and life viewpoint. It is either from an internal frame of reference, what we call ABOVE-DOWN-INSIDE-OUT (ADIO), also called, TOP-DOWN, or from an external frame of reference called OUTSIDE-IN-BELOW-UP (OIBU), also called, BOTTOM-UP. However human beings have a tendency to have a combination of both frames of references, at times, in order to construct a worldview that is most true to reality having universality of application and being life-like.

Chiropractic falls under the umbrella of ADIO. The initial condition of chiropractic's basic science is a universal principle of organization inherent to all E/matter, which supplies it properties and actions that maintains it in existence (Prin. 1). Therefore, the starting point of chiropractic's basic science is a universal principle intrinsic to all existence. From this initial principle, through deductive reasoning, we elaborate on the meaning, outcomes and manifestations of this one basic truth, which cascade into 32 subsequent principles. The instructive information provided by those principles is a solid bedrock platform on which chiropractic's blueprint is designed, ready to be used by its applied science through the art of chiropractic practice. Then through chiropractic philosophy, we understand that organization bespeaks intelligence. Rational logic follows and asserts that the cause of this universal principle of organization is a universal intelligence. It is a hard to vary philosophical explanation of the cause of the initial condition of chiropractic's basic science. We affirm that existence and life proceed from this universal principle of organization with its essential extension, the innate law of living things, down to the specific E/matter providing it with organized information/F internally to be expressed into multitudes of manifestations externally. Thus, the ADIO viewpoint embodies chiropractic philosophy. The chiropractic approach to life evidences the ADIO viewpoint and is only a part of it. There is much more to the ADIO viewpoint of life than chiropractic. Chiropractic addresses interference in transmission of innate impulses caused by vertebral subluxations (Prin. 29, 31a). The ADIO viewpoint is not part of chiropractic. However, chiropractic is part of the ADIO viewpoint. The ADIO viewpoint of life is consistent with chiropractic philosophy. It empowers practice members to make elegant choices for themselves in all aspects of their lives. For this reason, we educate everyone about the significance of having their spines and nerve system checked for vertebral subluxations on regular basis. We also show them how consistent it is with the ADIO viewpoint of life. In this way, human beings can subjectively and freely choose to avail themselves of chiropractic care.

One of the essentials of the ADIO viewpoint is the fact that there are absolutes in life as opposed to the OIBU viewpoint, which claims that everything is relative. While this may appear to be true, upon further observation it is an illusion that stems from the perspective of the individual part being separated from the whole. For example, you have a pot of water. The water molecules have the property of being fluid. Add a catalyst in the form of heat, say fire under the pot, and the universal principle of organization will organize the water molecules that have now acquired a different property and have morphed into gas. Do the opposite and refrigerate the water by removing heat, and now the universal principle of organization will organize the molecules of water providing them with the property of solid ice. Same electrons, protons and neutrons form the atoms of the water molecules. However, their velocities have been changed and they now have different actions as well as different properties provided by the universal principle of organization. The composition of a molecule of H_2O is always two atoms of hydrogen and one atom of oxygen regardless of its physical properties. It is an absolute and its formula is: $R_1 + R_2 \rightarrow \Delta E = P$.[31] The universal principle of organization (Prin. 1) is an absolute. The principle of time is an absolute (Prin. 6). The principle of cause and effect is an absolute (Prin. 17). The innate law of living things (Prin. 20) is an absolute. The limitation of structural E/matter (Prin. 24) is an absolute. The law of continuous supply and computation is an absolute (Prin. 33). Those principles and laws are not relative. Those principles and laws are absolute. They have universal applicability. They are no different from the universal law of gravitation, the laws of conservation, the laws of thermodynamics, etc.

Another essential of the ADIO viewpoint is the differentiation between absolute principles and the development of the relative educated intelligence over time. Absolutes do not change. Knowledge does change due to new information and the limitation of our educated intelligence, which is the capability of our educated brain to function (see lexicon). For example, principle 17 states that every effect has a cause and every cause has effects. This means that from the ADIO viewpoint the cause must be addressed if it is possible, as opposed to the OIBU approach which is to address effects with the objective to treat symptoms and diseases. The chiropractic objective is always about cause. Chiropractic is always about what is possible according to universal laws (Prin. 24). The foremost distinction between ADIO and OIBU is that the universal organizing principle, designed by a 100%/perfect universal intelligence, is superior to the continuously evolving educated intelligence. This means that the actual universal control of the universal principle of organization is the rule that governs the universe. The actual innate control of the innate law of living things is the rule that governs living organisms, including the human body. The best that educated control can do is to remove subluxations to restore transmission in the body in order to receive conducted innate information/F with innate-normal momentum. Chiropractic does just that by addressing exclusively the interference in transmission of innate impulses at the vertebral level for coordination of activities of all the parts of the body (Prin. 31a, 31b, 32) and it requires humility from the educated intelligence.

The original 1927 chiropractic textbook was written with the idea that chiropractic enclosed everything and that it was superior to religion, medicine and ethics. B.J. wrote specifically about it in his publication, *My Message Analyzed*.[32] Chiropractic consisted of answers to the physical, mental and spiritual ills of mankind. Chiropractic was the answer to getting sick people well in those days. Chiropractors never really knew about the ADIO worldview, as we understand it today. They were equating the ADIO viewpoint with chiropractic philosophy, stating that life flows from "Innate" above

---

31. Lessard, Claude. "Timed Out: Chiropractic." Self-Published, Claude Lessard, D.C. (2022) p. 39

32. Palmer, B.J., "My Message Analyzed."

in the brain, down to the body inside and out to the environment. However, it is the ADIO worldview that includes the chiropractic philosophy. The chiropractic approach to life evidences the ADIO viewpoint because it affects every human experience. It is life-like, and it has universal applicability. The ADIO worldview includes chiropractic. Chiropractic is only a portion of the ADIO viewpoint. The importance of this distinction is paramount to understanding the next section concerning poison, food, diet, exercise and hygiene, which are not part of the chiropractic objective. Chiropractic is not concerned with those aspects of life. The purpose of these topics is to have the student develop a deeper appreciation for the innate law that adapts, controls, and processes information/F and E/matter for use in the body, so that all parts of the body will have coordinated actions for mutual benefit (Prin. 23, 32), if it is possible according to universal laws (Prin. 24). Chiropractic philosophy explains why chiropractic, through the practice of its objective, addresses every facet of life through the correction of vertebral subluxations according to the principles of its basic science. Since the living body is regulated by body chemistry through the coordinated activities of all its parts controlled by the innate law, chiropractic directly relates to every facet of the human experience. The student is reminded that chiropractic is only about the restoration in transmission of innate impulses through the correction of vertebral subluxations. Nothing more. Nothing less. Nothing else.

One hundred years ago, there was no accreditation agency to regulate chiropractic colleges and universities and no state laws to govern the practice of chiropractic. Legislations came much later. Unfortunately, our collective educated intelligence in the 20th century was not developed and evolved to be able to "see" then what we now "see" today. The governing statutes, that rule the practice of chiropractic today, came to be enforced as a result of personal preferences from many lawmakers based on a limited understanding of what chiropractic really was one hundred years ago. It seems that confusing chiropractic philosophy with ADIO worldview was very common in those days. Then there were individuals who had an OIBU worldview and wanted to get sick people well, and even better than medicine could. Furthermore, many chiropractors were embracing the "one cause, one cure" idea and that chiropractic was the answer to all the ills of humankind. Today the practice of chiropractic is regulated by governmental laws that differ from State to State, which leaves the profession utterly divided, confused and adversarial. As we clarify the universal value of chiropractic's basic science, we are invited to choose what is right and not expedient based on universal truths rather that personal preferences. This is the motivation behind updating and re-writing the *1927 Chiropractic Textbook* from Ralph W. Stephenson, D.C. with the new information of the 21st century that provide us with a new lens to "see" today what we could not "see" one hundred years ago. Today, we only see what we can and we cannot yet see what will be seen one hundred years from now. That is how educated intelligence, which is the capability of the educated brain to function, evolves over time. What will remain the same is that chiropractic is a philosophy, science and art that is separate and distinct from everything else and inclusive of everyone. It is universally applicable and relatable to every bit of the human experience. Chiropractic is about life.

Articles 166 through 190 are written from the perspective of ADIO philosophy. Chiropractic does not address these issues, except that they act as penetrative information/F that requires adaptation from the innate law. Chiropractic addresses only the location, analysis and facilitation of the correction of vertebral subluxations (Prin. 31a, 31b), which restores the transmission of innate impulses (Prin. 29, 30) for coordination of activities of the parts of the body (Prin. 32).

ART. 166. POISON

The updated chiropractic definition of poison is any substance introduced into or manufactured within the living body in which the innate law cannot adapt or process for use in metabolism without breaking a universal law (Prin. 24). This definition can be found within the chiropractic lexicon.

ART. 167. THE POSSIBILITIES OF POISON

Poison possibilities are the distinctive ways in which poisons may occur. The following four possibilities are inclusive of any and every way that poisoning may occur:

1. Misplaced glandular products

2. Excess glandular products

3. Circulated glandular products

4. That which the innate law cannot process and use in the general metabolism of the body

Glandular products are only usable in the places that the innate law can process them according to universal laws (Prin. 24). If due to in-coordination of activities and these products are in any place where they should not be, they are poison.

In any part of the body for any given time, a specific level of the correct glandular products is required. If there is an excess of a glandular product, even in the proper systems of the body, it is a poison. It will affect the transport of the serous circulation as well.

If a misplaced glandular product is in a part of the body where it does not belong, it is a poison. From an ADIO viewpoint, the introduction of a product taken from one body and introduced into another body is a poison if it cannot be adapted and processed by the innate law.

Any substance in the body, whether glandular or not, which the innate law cannot process for use in metabolism is a poison. This includes both chemically active and inert substances. This fourth possibility will be explained fully in the following articles.

ART. 168. WHAT WE KNOW ABOUT POISONS

What our collective educated intelligence knows about poisons is the knowledge that tells us what substances are poisonous from accumulated experiences of people in general. What our collective educated intelligence knows about poison is from the lack of adaptability of the body to neutralize or counteract the substance involved. The Merrian-Webster dictionary defines poison as a substance that through its chemical action usually kills, injures, or impairs an organism. Something destructive or harmful. An object of aversion or abhorrence.

Educated intelligence with its accumulated knowledge thus far, knows that such a substance has the destroying property potential within it at all times. Carbolic acid, for example, is known to be a poison which will act in that deconstructive way. The collective educated intelligence continuously evolves and gains this knowledge by experience and observation. Educated intelligence does not know that a substance is poison, in actuality, until it is introduced into the body. However, educated intelligence has the general and useful knowledge of chemicals, which reveals that substances may act harmfully if taken into the body. Furthermore, by knowledge of chemicals, the collective educated intelligence might be able to compute which new chemicals may be poison according to their elementary compositions. Yet, this knowledge is limited according to the information available at the moment. Our collective educated intelligence only knows with certainty about the tested and proven poisonous substances when the innate law cannot adapt and process within the limitation of E/matter according to universal laws (Prin. 24).

ART. 169. WHAT WE DO NOT KNOW ABOUT POISONS

Our collective educated intelligence does not know that a substance is a poison until the innate law that controls the body cannot adapt and process a substance according to universal laws (Prin. 24). It has to be computed first and processed by the innate law, which then becomes an experience. It is through experiences that educated intelligence labels that particular substance a poison. Educated intelligence does not know if a new discovered chemical is poison until it is introduced in the body, whether inert or active.

This fact stresses that educated intelligence is truly inadequate in knowing with certainty all the substances that are poison to the body. It is only after the substance has been introduced into the body and its manifestation observed by the educated intelligence that we know for certain that it is a poison. Even as it is vital for our collective educated intelligence to accumulate knowledge to help us avoid poisons, this experiential fact crystallizes the importance to put our confidence in the 100%/perfect innate law and not educated intelligence, no matter how clever we are (Prin. 5, 22, 23, 25, 27, 32, 33).

ART. 170. HOW OUR COLLECTIVE EDUCATED INTELLIGENCE FOUND OUT ABOUT POISON SUBSTANCES

Educated knowledge of poisons is the sum total of human observation and experience as regard to the biological processes of substances by the innate law in adapting information/F and E/matter for use in the body (Prin. 23).

Our collective educated intelligence accumulates knowledge through observation, experimentation, study, and experience. We record information regarding substances and that is how it becomes human knowledge… of poisons in this instance.

With reference to biological processes of substances, it is the innate law that is the 100%/perfect innate software, which is normal, (Prin. 5, 22, 27, 33) that will adapt, through computation, information/F and E/matter of living things only if is possible according to universal laws (Prin. 23, 24). The function of the innate law is a continuous 100%/perfect computation moment by moment for as long as the body is alive without breaking a universal law (Prin. 21, 23, 24, 33). There are many factors involved in the innate processing of substances according to universal laws (genetics, quantity and quality of substances, previous exposures, etc.).

When I was three years old my parents discovered that tomatoes were noxious to my body. I developed what is called "urticaire" which is a poison elimination function in the form of inflammatory rash all over the body with extreme heat. However, what was a poison for my body was not a poison for my parents' bodies or my siblings' bodies. When I was 20 years old, I worked for a road maintenance company during our summer break and all the employees were instructed to be careful not to come in contact with poison ivy. Yet, there was a 50 year-old co-worker who had no problem with poison ivy. He even smeared it all over his arms and face without any reaction at all. His body possessed genetic properties and actions that allowed the adaptability of its E/matter to be less limited than most, regarding poison ivy.

Suffice to say that it is from the computation and processing of the 100%/perfect innate software that a substance will be classified as a poison by our collective educated intelligence because of a lack of adaptation by the innate law due to the limitation of E/matter (Prin. 24). It is therefore through the limitation of structural living E/matter that we come to know poison substances. Vertebral subluxations further increase the limitation of E/matter from its already genetic state due to a lack of coordination of activities of the body parts. This fact underscores once again the absolute importance to practice only the chiropractic objective. Our educated intelligence, which is the capability of our educated brain to function, is also subjected to the limitation of its E/matter. It is unreliable in regards to knowing everything there is to know about a substance that interacts with a particular body, at a particular moment, internally or externally. Only the 100%/perfect innate law can process that specific substance, moment by moment in accordance with universal laws (Prin. 24).

ART. 171. SENTIENT COMPUTATION OF BIOLOGICAL PROCESSES OF POISON

A poison is any substance introduced into or manufactured within the living body that the innate law cannot compute through adaptation of E/matter for use in the body without breaking a universal law. The innate law is a 100%/perfect software that can adapt universal information/F and living E/matter for use in the body only if it is possible to universal laws (Prin. 23, 24). Any substance that cannot be processed by the innate law for use in metabolism is a poison to that particular living body at that specific moment.

Our educated knowledge continually evolves over time. Yet the knowledge of poisons is limited to experience by the body or through laboratory experiments up to now. If a substance does not have the property of assimilability by the body of a living thing it will not be for use in that body. However, if the E/matter of a living body cannot be adapted due to its limitations at a determined moment, it may become adaptable at another moment in time. This means that a substance might be a poison for a living body only at a particular moment. For example, as a young child, I myself could not eat tomatoes without manifesting severe "urticaire". I almost died. Tomatoes were poison to my body. However, I found out when I was in my fifties that I could eat tomatoes without any problem at all. Tomatoes are not a poison to me any longer. Perhaps this is due to being under regular chiropractic care since 1974 and now my body has less limitation of its E/matter that had been once increased by the presence of vertebral subluxations.

The fact remains that it is the normal function of the 100%/perfect innate law to adapt universal information/F and E/matter, through sentient computation, moment by moment, for use in the body in accordance to universal laws (Prin. 23, 24, 27). For this reason, our collective educated intelligence, which is the capability of our educated brain to function, evolves over time and our knowledge of poisons grows. Along with its will and memory components, our collective educated intelligence can keep this information into a record of poison substances that we can definitely avoid.

All things belong in the universe. Due to the limitation of E/matter and time, it is the innate law that ultimately determines if a substance is a poison for a specific living organism moment by moment. It behooves us to continuously practice the chiropractic objective displaying universal values. As we facilitate the correction of vertebral subluxations, we participate in the restoration of the transmission of innate impulses, which in turn satisfies the principle of coordination (Prin. 29, 30, 31a, 31b, 32).

Dr. Claude Lessard

REVIEW QUESTIONS FOR ARTICLES 162 - 171

1. What is afferent poisoning of serum?
2. What is unsoundness from excess water serum?
3. What is unsoundness from insufficient water serum?
4. Concerning the serous circulation, what is that chiropractic claims as its discovery?
5. What is the updated chiropractic definition of poison?
6. Name and explain the four possibilities of poison.
7. According to chiropractic, how is a substance determined a poison?

ART. 172. SOME ACCUMULATED KNOWLEDGE OF POISONS

Any substance that is adaptable, or that the living body can be adapted to, by the innate law for use in the living body, is a food (Prin. 23, 24). Philosophically this is true even in the case of medications. For example, medicine is a substance given with the intent to "stimulate" or "inhibit" certain functions of the living body. It is Outside-In-Below-Up (OIBU) thinking. Sometimes it stimulates, sometimes it inhibits and sometimes it is rejected by the body. This becomes clear to us through observation and tests at that particular moment. It is solely dependent upon whether the medication administered is adaptable, and the limitation of E/matter of that unique living body at that particular time. Drugs are OIBU and always cause side effects, which are an indication of the stress that they cause the body as poisonous substances. The innate law will adapt information/F (in this case the medication) and E/matter (in this case that unique living body) only if it is possible without breaking a universal law because the innate law is limited by the limitation of E/matter (Prin. 24).

Some substances, that our educated intelligence calls foods, are sometimes poisons due to their additives cancer producing capabilities.

Some substances that are good for one person may be poison to another.

Some substances may be foods for a person at one point, and poisons for the same person at another time.

Anything introduced into the body that is not adaptable or that the body cannot be adapted to, is a poison.

Any substance introduced into the living body, whether it is a poison or not, depends upon whether it can be adapted, or that the living E/matter can be adapted to it, for use in the body, by the innate law without breaking a universal law (Prin. 23, 24). If it can, it is a food. If it cannot, it is a poison. If the information/F introduced into the body is a substance that is useful to that unique living body, at that particular moment in time, it is food. If it is not useful, it is poison.

ART. 173. FOOD

Food is any substance ingested into the body, which when digested and otherwise prepared, supplies wholesome nutrition to the tissue cells. The necessary elements for metabolism are provided by the external environment, or manufactured by the body glands and organs. From an ADIO perspective, these necessities are made known to us by natural hunger, cravings and desire. Our collective educated intelligence is very limited and the innate law with its integral processing (100%/perfect) is so capable, that it benefits us to favor those natural hunger, cravings and desires rather than to determine, through educated intelligence, what we think is best.

Given the necessary materials, the innate law will adapt, codify and process them in any combination required for metabolism only if it is possible according to universal laws (Prin. 24). Given the unnecessary materials, the innate law will codify them as rejects that will go through the elimination systems to be excreted.

When prevented from receiving necessary materials for metabolism, the innate law, through body economy will process the amount of what is already stored until depleted. If the situation persists some tissues will become unsound. If given too much food to the body, the innate law will adapt and process information/F along with E/matter to excrete the unneeded excess of materials, only if it is possible according to universal laws (Prin. 24). If a person constantly overeats, or has vertebral subluxations, there will come point where the elimination systems of the body will be overworked and will be limited from excreting normally, thus the excess materials will become overstored in the cells or become poisons that will make the cells unsound.

This fact underscores the necessity for regular chiropractic care and to understand that our educated intelligence cannot regulate and determine our nutritional needs. We just do not know the body's minimum or maximum daily requirements. These educated numbers are only "average." Environment, culture, genetics, climate, daily circumstances, and the uniqueness of each individual body moment to moment are of such a magnitude as to really baffle the educated control regarding nutritional requirements moment by moment.

Suffice to say that the ADIO understanding of nutrition is to follow individual natural hunger, individual natural cravings, individual natural thirst, individual natural desire and individual natural restraint. "Individual" was mentioned because one can only know those hunger, cravings, thirst, desires or restraints for oneself and for no one else from an ADIO viewpoint. Chiropractic philosophy encourages the individual to get their spine and nerve system checked regularly. Chiropractic's basic science provides the possibility of restoration of normal transmission of innate impulses for the individual. The art of chiropractic applies principles of its basic science that provide the instructions necessary to have their vertebral subluxations corrected (Prin. 23, 24, 27, 31a, 31b).

Since vertebral subluxations further increase the limitation of E/matter of the body, it is important for the student to recognize the unique and immense responsibility of the chiropractor to practice exclusively the chiropractic objective in order to serve people regardless of any other needs they may have that can be served by other professionals. Chiropractic is separate and distinct from everything else and inclusive of everyone.

ART. 174. DIET

Dieting, as commonly understood, is not consistent with chiropractic philosophy. Dieting is an educated choice attempting to control or regulate the functions of the body. It is determining what the nutrition of the body should be at that moment. It is OIBU. Dieting is not chiropractic.

Merriam-Webster Dictionary defines *diet* as:

> **1a:** Food and drink regularly provided or consumed
>
> **1b:** Habitual nourishment
>
> **1c:** The kind and amount of food prescribed for a person or animal for a special reason
>
> **1d:** A regimen of eating and drinking sparingly so as to reduce one's weight

From these definitions it is commonly understood that dieting is a prescribed regimen of food for some therapeutic reason. According to the principles of its basic science, chiropractic is strictly non-therapeutic. Therefore, dieting is not consistent with chiropractic philosophy, or chiropractic's basic science, or the art of chiropractic. It is reserved to the nutritionist to deal with dieting, not chiropractors.

Prescription is a therapeutic procedure used in the medical model of treating symptoms and diseases. Chiropractic does attempt to judge medical procedures or their intents. Sometimes dieting produces the therapeutic desired effects, and sometimes it does not. It is OIBU and it is an arbitrary attempt at regulating the metabolism of the body, which is under the direct control of the 100%/perfect innate law. Chiropractic is about cause and not effect.

From an ADIO perspective, anyone who eats according to natural hunger, craving, thirst and desire will easily eat appropriate quantities and qualities of natural food available within her environment.

This underscores the importance to practice the chiropractic objective displaying universal values so that, through the correction of vertebral subluxations, the restoration of transmission of innate impulses is accomplished and the limitation of E/matter is not any further increased. After all, educated intelligence, which is the capability of the educated brain to function, has limitations of the E/matter of its physical brain (Prin. 24). Our collective educated intelligence is not equipped to dictate what it thinks what food the body requires at any given moment. It is OIBU. Only the individual who acts on its natural hunger, natural thirst, natural cravings and natural desires is responsible to nourish his own body in a natural way. That is ADIO.

ART. 175. GOOD EDUCATED CHOICE OF NUTRITION BASED ON NATURAL HUNGER, NATURAL CRAVINGS, NATURAL THIRST, AND NATURAL DESIRES IS ADIO

When the body assimilates the food materials according to natural hunger or thirst, the innate law will adapt, code and process it for use in the body in any combination if it is possible according to universal laws (Prin. 23, 24).

Our collective educated intelligence should not presume to determine the calories or to determine the materials, which the human body requires for metabolism. This presumption stems from OIBU thinking. Objective chiropractors realize that it is the individual's responsibility to be informed and to select materials for himself according to his natural hunger or thirst. It is important to note that a good educated choice is understood as being as natural as possible. It stems from ADIO thinking. For this to occur, coordination of activities of body parts, including the educated brain, is paramount. It points to the necessity to have vertebral subluxations correction for normal transmission of innate impulses (Prin. 28, 29, 30, 31a, 31b, 32, 33). However, even with normal transmission of innate impulses, our collective educated is not positioned to know what is good or what is bad for another. What is good for one person may be poison for another *(See Art. 172)*.

Nutritional hygiene is good educated habits coming out from good educated choices. It is eating and drinking according to natural hunger and natural thirst. It is simply the restoration of natural conditions of the external environment through educated control, which is the activity of the educated brain. It is "listening" to the body's natural urges moment to moment. It is ADIO. Even with normal transmission of innate impulses, the best we can do is usually an educated guess regarding the materials that are required by the human body. The best we can do, as objective chiropractors along with practicing the chiropractic objective, is to encourage our practice members to think from an ADIO viewpoint. They can choose foods and drinks according to their natural hunger and thirst, so that they can learn to make good educated choices for themselves. We must remember, however, that ultimately it is not so much what we do to our body in consuming foods and drinks but what our body does for using those foods and drinks that matters. Elegant choices are important when it comes to issues of foods and drinks. In the following article we will address some of the factors that influence our educated choices of foods and drinks.

Dr. Claude Lessard

ART. 176. THE PARADOX OF THE COLLECTIVE EDUCATED CONTROL OF ALWAYS CHOOSING ABOVE-DOWN-INSIDE-OUT VERSUS SOMETIMES CHOOSING OUTSIDE-IN-BELOW-UP

These two viewpoints need not being antagonistic toward one another. In chiropractic, the initial conception was that ADIO was opposed to OIBU. Today, we understand that it is not the case any longer. With today's knowledge, we recognize the need for both (at times) and how to integrate them without any conflict. Here we come face to face with a paradox. First of all, the chiropractic objective is, "the location, analysis and facilitation of the correction of vertebral subluxations for an innate-normal transmission of innate impulses." Nothing more. Nothing less. Nothing else. Period. The student should note that it is the restoration of normal transmission of innate impulses for the coordination of activities of body parts that is the aim of the chiropractic objective, not the function of the tissue cell (Prin. 32, 33). It is for this reason that the chiropractic model is separate and distinct from everything, including the medical model, the aim of which is to stimulate or to inhibit the function of the tissue cell. Yet, sometimes it may be necessary to have a medical intervention to alter the functions of the body in order to "help" the body go through unusual emergencies (broken bones, burned skin, tooth decay, etc.). On the other hand, chiropractic care is always necessary for the body to receive its innate-normal transmission of innate impulses for the coordination of activities of all its parts. To be free of vertebral subluxations is always vital to the purpose of the innate law, which is to keep the material of the body alive. It is up to each person to use their educated brain and educated intelligence to always choose to have chiropractic care and to sometimes to choose to have medical emergency procedures when absolutely necessary. Hopefully the practice member is a person who has a good understanding of the ADIO philosophy of life through knowing and internalizing the principles of chiropractic's basic science.

For that to occur, it is the responsibility of the chiropractors to educate their practice members about the principles of chiropractic and their universal values, and to teach them both, ADIO and OIBU approaches. The mission of the chiropractic profession is the specific task of increasing the awareness of the universal values of chiropractic to the whole world.

It is meant for the person to adhere to the principles without wavering to the external pressures and influences of life circumstances. You either follow universal principles or you follow whatever the world proclaims you ought to do based on personal and preferential recommendations. Remember that, ultimately, only the individual is capable determining and choosing what is best for him or her alone (that is the reason why everyone signs terms of acceptance in an objective chiropractor's office, and in a medical establishment, everyone signs waivers of responsibilities regarding medical treatments and interventions). We must understand that our collective educated intelligence is absolutely inadequate with regard to coordinating the activities of the parts of the human body. It is only the normal innate law of living things and its function (Prin. 27), which is the 100%/perfect innate software that adapts, codes and processes information/F and E/matter (Prin. 23), that is continually supplied by the universal law of continuous supply and computation (Prin. 33), that is always controlling all of the functions of the body and for coordination of activities of its parts and for use in metabolism (Prin. 23), only if it is possible according to universal laws (Prin. 24). Of course, this again underscores the importance of being free of vertebral subluxations (Prin. 31a, 31b) to restore the transmission of innate impulses in order to have maximum efficiency of every phase of our life (including choice making). Chiropractic care is paramount to effectively make elegant choices for one's wellbeing. It boils down to actually do the very best that is possible under the circumstance with regard to choosing to do what is required for the individual's wellbeing. For chiropractors, it is the responsibility of every chiropractor to practice exclusively the chiropractic objective and to teach the principles of chiropractic's basic science persistently using chiropractic philosophy, over and over again in as many ways as possible. If practice members internalize and own those principles, it can provide them with knowledge and fortify people with the wisdom necessary to make elegant choices regarding their wellbeing.

According to the instructions of the principle of chiropractic's basic science, it is not within the scope of chiropractic practice to tell people what to do with their nutrition, exercise, posture, attitude or sleep. Those facets of living are necessary and are attended as being the objectives of nutritionists, therapists, trainers and life coaches. The chiropractic objective is absolutely unique, separate and distinct from everything else because the chiropractic objective addresses a cause of interference of transmission of innate impulses, directly or indirectly (Prin. 23, 29, 31a, 31b, 32, 33).

Natural hunger and thirst are dependent upon coordination of activities of all the parts of the body (including the educated brain) and their sound vitality. Innate-normal computation, coding and processing of information/F and E/matter for use in the body, by the innate law, is dependent upon innate-normal transmission through conductivity of innate impulses and through radiation of innate rays. Chiropractic addresses the transmission of innate impulses, exclusively, through the practice of its objective, which is derived from the 33 principles of chiropractic's basic science.

It is the innate law that governs all the functions of the living body, including its nourishment. The innate law is a 100%/perfect software that continually adapts, computes, codes and processes information/F and E/matter for use in the body (Prin. 23, 33). From an ADIO perspective, our educated control being dependent upon normal transmission, serves as a cooperative function to selectively assimilate foods and water from natural hunger, natural thirst, natural cravings and natural desires.

Foods and water introduced into the body when not required are poisons. Any artificially processed food and water are poison for they are not natural.

The principles of chiropractic's basic science allow us to be consistently aware that most things in the universe are not permanent. Rocks are continually broken down to their most stable atomic state; the pages of this book will thin out, turn yellow, and tear; living things will eventually die and decay. Only the elemental electrons, protons, and neutrons of E/matter, along with quarks and other fundamental particles, including their information, will always be continually maintained in existence due to the universal principle of organization (Prin. 1). While the structural systems do change, their fundamental constituents stay unchanged giving rise to the laws of conservation. We observe with crystal clarity that the universal principle of organization is a fundamental truth that is the foundation of universal laws that is entirely responsible for E/matter to be maintained in existence perpetually. The universal principle of organization puts incredible pressure on everything in the universe: on all that has happened from the beginning of time and all that will happen from now on forward. The universal principle of organization is the principle that organizes the information/F of the orbits of planets, governs the expansion of the universe. It organizes the information/F supplying our bodies, organizes the information/F of electrical and electronic currents in our computer devices, controls the adapted inner functions for the metabolism of living organisms through its essential extension, which is the innate law. It organizes information/F that generate the clouds in the sky, the waves in the ocean, the fluid molten rock in the center of our planet. Its ability to organize E/matter extends even beyond what actually occurs in the universe to include limitation of structural E/matter that would restrain certain processing of information/F for biological adaptation. Whatever the universal laws prevent from happening cannot ever occur, regardless of the effort exerted to make it happen. As an example, you cannot create E/matter from no E/matter, because the universal principle of organization continually organizes information/F that provides properties and actions to E/matter, thus maintaining it in existence (Prin. 1). The E/matter of the universe is conserved, never created nor destroyed. You can only reorganize E/matter in ways that have the property of copy-ability. You can only construct that which can be copied. It already exists in principle. "You cannot give what you do not already have." You cannot invent what cannot be invented. The universal principle of organization is the fundamental explanation for the breaking down of E/matter into its most stable state of elementary components such as atoms. Under the universal principle of organization, dense structures of atoms, like boulders, are continually altered by their synergy with their external environment that brings about breakdown changes in their structural forms. Unless something were to step in to restore this breakdown, as in the adaptation of living organisms, the structural E/matter will eventually decay or crumble. The higher the level of complexities of the structural form, the more difficult it is to maintain it whole over time. It requires flexibility through adaptability. It is living things that have these properties of flexibility and adaptability, due to the intrinsic innate law within every living thing. A human being has the property of self-healing. A boulder does not. A person will certainly die at one point, however the human species may survive for much longer that the boulder can. For this reason, chiropractic is only about what is possible, which is the restoration of transmission of innate impulses through the correction of vertebral subluxations. It is the momentum of the transmission of these conducted information/F that maintains the sequences of instructions in the form of innate impulses for coordination of activities of body parts that chiropractic addresses. Nothing more. Nothing less. Nothing else.

ART. 177. EXERCISE

Exercise is the natural movements of the body and its parts to facilitate adaptation by the innate law. The law of continuous supply and computation provides the necessary information/F to the body. For this reason, the objective of chiropractic is to correct vertebral subluxation for the innate-normal transmission of information/F that have been adapted and coded into innate impulses.

From the ADIO viewpoint, natural exercise comes from making elegant choices in discernment and derives a natural tiredness as opposed to over exercising which produces a fatigue or exhaustion.

The rule regarding exercise, from an ADIO viewpoint, is for the individual to follow guidance in the form of urges or promptings of the body for natural movements to obtain normal adaptation by the innate law (Prin. 23, 27).

The body is designed to be active promoting adaptation by the innate law. Physical therapists, trainers and physical education teachers are people whose specific job is to help people to exercise. Chiropractors, on the other hand, insure that there are no vertebral subluxations that interfere with the transmission of innate impulses for coordination of activities of body parts, exclusively. In this way natural exercise can be better discerned by each individual person, free of vertebral subluxations, in order to promote adaptation.

ART. 178. HYGIENE

Hygiene, from an ADIO point of view, is the restoration of natural environment conditions, which have been altered by civilization. In many instances, where it is impossible to restore natural conditions, compensation must be made. Civilization is the necessary sacrifices that individuals must make regarding personal values in order to live in communities, to avoid infringing upon the rights of others, to give service that is coordinated. Therefore, the practice of the chiropractic objective fosters universal values for the coordination of activities of all the parts of the body facilitating the correction of vertebral subluxations to compensate for the many difficulties that our collective educated control distorted. Civilization, which embraces mostly the OIBU viewpoint, is necessary at the cost of moving away from natural choices and the ADIO viewpoint. However, as human beings endowed with the most competent organs of environmental adaptation of any living creatures, the educated brain, it is possible to embrace the ADIO viewpoint and compensate for what we lose in naturalness. This is possible by educationally restoring naturalness to the best of our abilities. The student is reminded that chiropractic is always about what is possible. For the objective chiropractors, this means to exclusively practice the chiropractic objective displaying universal values in order to restore transmission of innate impulses through the facilitation of the correction of vertebral subluxations. This is the meaning of hygiene from an ADIO perspective.

ART. 179. THE POISONS OF ENVIRONMENT

Extremely adverse environmental conditions for the human body are important in the study of the adaptability of the body. They affect adaptation by presenting detrimental conditions from OIBU that make it more difficult to achieve due to further limiting the genetic limitation of E/matter (Prin. 24).

Poor environmental conditions affect the adaptability of the body due to limitation of E/matter. This is exacerbated if vertebral subluxations exist, since vertebral subluxations further limit the limitation of E/matter. In our studies of environmental poisoning, the serous circulation is the main factor in the consideration of innate-normal serous flow of serum.

Environmental conditions can make adaptation extremely difficult and impossible in many cases, even for a person without vertebral subluxations. We do not know to what extent the environment is a factor in the cause of a lack of adaptation. The only responsibility that a chiropractor can fulfill is to make sure that there are no vertebral subluxations so that the body can adapt to the environment to the best of its abilities, with less limitation of E/matter due to the restoration of transmission of innate impulses for the individual. It is important to educate people about the ADIO and the OIBU viewpoints of life. If we chiropractors follow the instructions of the 33 principles of chiropractic's basic science, displaying universal values, we will be using them as our GPS to make error corrections that will keep us on course rather than developing more OIBU solutions to problems that stems from OIBU thinking.

ART. 180. WATER, AIR, SUNLIGHT, AND CLIMATE AS ENVIRONMENT FACTORS

Climate change is part of the natural adaptation of planet earth. Our planet is vitalistic, therefore its components are vitalistic as well. The innate law of living things is intrinsic to our living planet. There is the innate law of the planet that governs every bit of all the bodies of living things, from a blade of grass all the way up to a human being. Planet earth is bursting with life and gazillions living organisms that are constantly adapting to environmental changes. From a universal organizing principle (Prin. 1), just the facts that the planet rotates on its tilted 23.4° axis at 1000 miles per hour, taking 24 hours for one full rotation; that it is orbiting around the sun at 66,000 miles per hour, taking 365 days for one full rotation, giving us spring, summer, fall and winter seasons; that the entire solar system orbits around its galaxy called the milky way at 500,000 miles per hour taking 225,000,000 years for one full rotation[33] truly reveals that we do not know very much about the cause of climate change. Yet, artificial living can have an impact on climate as we see the dwindling of rainforests and polluting of our

---
33. "Earth and the Solar System" science.nasa.gov/earth/facts June 2024

atmosphere. Hopefully, a person's body with coordination of activities (without vertebral subluxations) will have a better functioning educated brain to use as an effective tool to make elegant choices for the external environment.

Understanding the ADIO point of view, we can assuredly prove that the universal principle of organization does organize information/F that supplies properties and actions to all E/matter to maintain it in existence (Prin. 1) as the initial condition of chiropractic's basic science. We can also prove that the innate law of living things is intrinsic to all living E/matter and governs all of its activities, including the innate impulses for voluntary actions that have been tinctured (modified) by the educated brain into educated impulses. For this reason, the conclusion of the 33 principles of chiropractic's basic science describes its objective, displaying universal values, as being the location, analysis and facilitation of the correction of vertebral subluxation for an innate-normal transmission of the innate impulses of the body.

Of course, all species of life contribute to the wellbeing of its habitat as they stand out as having a great propensity for flexibility due to having the property of adaptability. Living things have the ability to express the five signs of life (Prin. 18) and self-healing. For example, bacteria have lived billions of years on earth almost unchanged. Their sequences of instructions are adapted by the innate law and are coded for how to construct a bacterium out of universal information/F and fundamental elements, (the DNA of every bacterial cell). This DNA molecule is the central unique sequence of instruction of any cell. It's a string of chemicals, called genes. It is the instructive information/F of these genes that have been maintained essentially the same over such a long period of time. Yet, structures of boulders on earth have changed dramatically over this long period of time. Continents have been transformed and reorganized, by the universal principle of organization, within the hot molten center of the planet through inner movements (Prin. 14, 15). Our planet still reveals the signs of bacterial activity of millions of years ago as in fossil carbon. Even plant materials continually transform our atmosphere through photosynthesis, processing light and converting it into chemistry. Human beings also reconstruct the environment in ways that were not known before humans existed, as they are one of the effects of the development of civilization. Issues like water, air, sunlight, and climate change are environmental effects of many factors, including civilization. One hundred years ago, when Ralph Stephenson, D.C. wrote his chiropractic textbook, the ground water and the air were certainly less polluted. These issues are human issues and not chiropractic issues. Chiropractic addresses only vertebral subluxations. These issues are mentioned here so that we understand that they play a part in the development of educated intelligence, which is the capability of the educated brain to function, and its accumulation of knowledge.

Human beings have the responsibility to be good steward of our planet in a way that is dictated by our conscious awareness due to our organs of adaptation and also the 100%/perfect innate software called the innate law of living things.

Our call as chiropractors is to practice exclusively the chiropractic objective, displaying universal values, in order to facilitate coordination of activities in the body. With an innate-normal transmission of innate impulses for coordination of activities of all the parts of the body, everyone may be better equipped to choose what is right for the planet in their own unique way and be responsible steward of our planet.

ART. 181. FOOD AS AN ENVIRONMENTAL FACTOR

Food that has been cultivated by chemical fertilizers, processed and loaded with preservatives or artificial coloring may poison a body of lowered natural genetic resistance. It will poison the serous circulation. It is derived from an OIBU viewpoint. Natural pure food that is coming from an ADIO viewpoint is more beneficial for the body so that the information/F it contains will supply the best material to be processed to benefit all the parts of the body for metabolism. As chiropractors, our job is to practice exclusively the chiropractic objective, which is derived from the 33 principles of chiropractic's basic science, and to teach people about ADIO and OIBU viewpoints.

Dr. Claude Lessard

REVIEW QUESTIONS FOR ARTICLES 172 - 181

1. Why is medication poison?
2. What is food?
3. When is food a poison?
4. How is a substance determined as food?
5. Is dieting consistent with chiropractic philosophy?
6. How do we know what food to eat at any given moment?
7. What is the cause of unnatural hunger and thirst?
8. Should chiropractors regulate the diet of their practice members?
9. Should chiropractors regulate the exercise of their practice members?
10. From an ADIO point of view, what is the definition of hygiene?
11. As chiropractors, what is the meaning of hygiene?
12. What are the possibilities of environmental poisoning?
13. What property do living things have regarding resistance to environmental factors?
14. Do human beings influence climate change?
15. Explain water supply as environmental factor.
16. Explain food as environmental factor.
17. What is the property that a substance must have to be classified as food?
18. Why is natural food beneficial to the body?
19. What is the responsibility of a chiropractor relative to people?

ART. 182. AIR AS ENVIRONMENTAL FACTOR

Air that is polluted with chemicals (OIBU) or that is imbalanced as regards to oxygen or carbon dioxide or other essential elements is an external invasive information/F that may cause a vertebral subluxation if it overcomes the internal resistance of the body. Effluvia of dead things is unfit for the human organism due limitation of E/matter. It is noxious gases and chemicals to the human body as it has limited adaptability. Our special sense organs are useful to warn us through smell, touch, sight or taste of such substances as long as they have no interference in transmission of innate impulses and that they are sound. This underscores the importance of chiropractors to practice the chiropractic objective to restore transmission of innate impulses through the correction of vertebral subluxations.

ART. 183. CLIMATE AS A FACTOR OF ENVIRONMENT

Climate, food, diet, water, and exercise do participate into the ADIO viewpoint as environmental factors. The innate law will have to adapt the universal information/F of the environmental factors for use in the body so that all the parts of the body will have coordination of actions (Prin. 23). They are external information/F that may invade the body and overcome its internal resistance. They may cause vertebral subluxations. However, these environmental factors are of no concern to chiropractic. They have no influence whatsoever regarding the chiropractic objective, which is exclusively, the location, analysis, and facilitation of the correction of the vertebral subluxation for an innate-normal transmission of innate impulses. It is absolutely important for the student to understand and to promote that chiropractic is separate and distinct from everything else and is inclusive of everyone.

Adverse climate can poison a body with a lowered natural resistance due to vertebral subluxations. The natural external environment is loaded with external invasive universal information/F that are deconstructive toward structural E/matter (Prin. 26). Those invasions need to be adapted by the innate law for use in the body and for coordination of activities of all its parts, to keep the body within innate-normal balance without causing harm to the body and that, only if it is possible according to universal laws (Prin. 23, 24, 27). Chiropractic addresses exclusively the correction of vertebral subluxations and, as such, contributes to positive survival values (ADIO), even though these environmental factors are outside our control. Environmental chemicals are external invasive information/F that the innate law must adapt in order to maintain balance in the body. It is imperative that human beings use their educated intelligence to choose wisely their intake of substances based on the ADIO viewpoint, which is the intake of natural materials with positive survival values for the innate law to adapt for use in the body. This innate adaptation will always require an innate-normal momentum of transmission of innate impulses, which underscores the importance of practicing the chiropractic objective exclusively.

ART. 184. HYGIENE AND SANITATION AS ENVIRONMENTAL FACTORS

Poor hygiene and deficient sanitation can poison the body with a lowered natural genetic resistance from vertebral subluxations, by further increasing the limitation of E/matter thus decreasing its level of adaptability, making it less adaptable by the innate law (Prin. 23, 24). From an ADIO viewpoint, it behooves the chiropractor to choose to practice the chiropractic objective exclusively for the restoration of the momentum for innate-normal transmission of innate impulses facilitating the process of a vertebral adjustment by the innate law (Prin. 31a, 31b).

Dr. Claude Lessard

ART. 185. EFFLUVIA AS AN ENVIRONMENTAL FACTOR

Effluvia is gases from putrid, decomposing and decaying organic E/matter that can poison the serous circulation, being an external invasive information/F that overcomes the internal resistance of the body, that may cause vertebral subluxations due to the limitation of E/matter. The toxicity of effluvia requires adaptation that is not possible without breaking a universal law (Prin. 24). Therefore, from an ADIO perspective, our special senses warn us to stay away or to move away from such poisonous gases.

ART. 186. GERMS AS A FACTOR OF ENVIRONMENT

Germs are living organisms that are governed by the same innate law that governs the human body. Essentially germs participate in the ecological system of planet Earth for its vitality and soundness. Some germs are necessary for human life, for nutritional value and to maintain the material of the human body in a innate-normal state of adaptability. The body develops from a seed that will fertilize a suitable host cell that will germinate and grow. Some germs are airborne. Some germs are found in water, and all living organism. Germs are part and parcel of the living environment and are adapted by the innate law for their own purposes, mostly as scavengers to clean up the environment. However, some germs can poison a body of lowered natural genetic resistance from vertebral subluxations. If the body's internal resistance is not compromised by a further increase of limitation of E/matter due to vertebral subluxations, the innate law will adapt, code and process the information/F and materials of germs (viruses and bacteria), if it is possible according to universal laws, for the benefit of all the parts of the body for coordination of activities including metabolism (Prin. 21, 23, 24).

The more civilization progresses on the evolutionary spectrum, the more the world is moving further away from its natural state. The advancement of humanity comes as a result of educated discoveries that are constructed into knowledge for the unfolding of the species. In the 21st century, the world contains an abundance of external invasive information/F that includes germs of all kinds. Some are from natural causes (ADIO) and possess constructive survival values. They are necessary for life to be sustained on Earth. Some are from artificial causes (OIBU) and possess deconstructive survival values. If they are in great numbers and their actions penetrate the body, overcoming its internal resistance, germs can harm living tissues. Their impact, as penetrative invasive information/F (see lexicon), can cause a vertebral subluxation if they overcome the internal resistance of the body. In turn, the vertebral subluxation will lower the internal natural genetic resistance of the body even more, further increasing the limitation of E/matter, directly or indirectly (Prin. 31a). Since germs can be penetrative invasive agents, they can cause vertebral subluxations and lowered natural genetic resistance may happen simultaneously with vertebral subluxations. However, as there are billions of cycles going on at the same time in the body, chiropractic maintains that the vertebral subluxation came first (Prin. 31a). This is consistent with the principles of chiropractic's basic science asserting that as the body expresses the information/F of the organizing principle (Prin. 13, 20), the body is maintained alive (Prin. 21). As the nerve system conducts innate-normal transmission of innate impulses for coordination of activities (Prin. 28) and as normal innate rays/waves radiate or oscillate from within the tissue cell for metabolism, the body receives its innate-normal momentum of innate information/F (Prin. 27), being vested with an innate-normal natural genetic resistance, according to its limitation of E/matter (Prin. 24). Chiropractic addresses only restoration in transmission of innate impulses through the correction of vertebral subluxations. Chiropractic does not address radiation or oscillation of innate rays/waves.

ART. 187. PARASITES

In the 1920s, parasites were thought to be absolutely negative and totally worthless. They did not belong. Today, however, with new information and knowledge we know that parasites stimulate the immune system of the host to produce chemicals using specific combination of organs and glands that will eradicate the parasite. Those specific chemicals also provide something necessary for the host in order to deal with its environment at that specific moment. [34] Depending upon the moment-by-moment circumstances, it is necessary for the body to deal with the stressors that are involved at specific times. Some body chemistry can only come about from unusual stimulants. It is the paradox of life. Parasites are of that unusual kind.

Parasites are organisms that are governed by the same innate law that governs all living things, including the human body. Therefore, the innate law adapts the information/F of the material of those parasites for use in the body only if it is possible according to universal laws (Prin. 20, 23, 24). It is always the limitation of E/matter that is the determining factor regarding its adaptability and never the innate law, which is 100%/perfect (Prin. 22). Since our educated knowledge is limited and dependent upon the information available, what we can be certain of, is that the innate law is a 100%/perfect innate software that governs every bit of living tissues, including parasites (Prin. 20, 22, 33). Therefore, since vertebral subluxations further increase the natural genetic limitation of living the living body (Prin. 24, 31a), it is important to continually practice the chiropractic objective.

Parasites feed upon the materials of their host. They do not thrive upon dead materials or waste E/matter of their host. They feed upon living tissues and good materials to survive. They do not feed on dead tissues as scavengers do, but require good food materials intended for the metabolism of the host. Thus, the innate law uses the immune system of the host to begin the production of chemistry that will exterminate the parasite according to the limits of adaptation of the host. Once again, remember that the 100%/perfect innate law (Prin. 22) is the same in the parasite, and the host. Only the innate law can process information/F and E/matter of both, host and parasite, to keep moment-by-moment everything balanced within the body of living organisms according to universal laws (Prin. 24) for all living things. It is implied in the same way regarding the innate law of the cell, the innate law of the organ, the innate law of the system and the innate law of the body, the innate law of all living things, the innate law of the life of the planet. Complete balance of motion (Prin. 15) within living organisms is dependent upon the information/F of the innate law, all according to their own particular limitations of E/matter (Prin. 20, 23, 24, 27).

The student may wonder if there is a hierarchy within living organisms. The answer is affirmative. The balance of living motion within the organism is directly proportional to its level of adaptability. If the adaptability of the body of the host is greater than the body of the parasite, the parasite will not survive and it will be eliminated through the excretory system of the host. If the adaptability of the parasite is greater that the host, imbalance of motion will be manifested by the host and deconstructive survival values will ensue. Since the innate law never injures or deconstructs the material of the structures in which it works (Prin. 25), it is clear that it is the lack of adaptability of E/matter of the parasite that causes the parasite to die. The function of the innate law is to always adapt information/F and E/matter only if it is possible according to universal laws (Prin. 23, 24).

---

34. Buckingham, L.J., & Ashby, B. (2022) Coevolutionary Theory of Hosts and Parasites. "Journal of Evolutionary Biology", 35, 205-224. DOI: 10.111/jeb.13981

Dr. Claude Lessard

ART. 188. EPIDEMICS, ENDEMICS, AND PANDEMICS

Epidemics, endemics and pandemics are the spreading of adverse conditions that may include extreme weather change, air or water pollution, including germs, bacteria and viruses. These events are penetrative information/F that can produce deconstructive survival values to the body of those who lack adaptability due to lowered natural genetic resistance from limitation of E/matter (Prin. 24) that has been, directly or indirectly, further induced and increased by vertebral subluxation (Prin. 31a). It underscores the importance for chiropractors to practice the chiropractic objective in order to restore the transmission of innate impulses for coordination of activities.

Most of the adverse conditions are often caused by an adverse environment that has been deconstructed by human beings as a result of artificially altering the environment to a point of reactionary consequences. For example, the excessive cutting of trees in the Amazon and in other areas of the world causes an imbalance of climate that promotes an excessive breeding of germs, insects and anaerobic organisms. Air and water pollution due to chemical residuals of factories and mechanical transportation have reactionary consequences on the environment, making it unnatural and unlivable at times. Chiropractic does not address those adverse conditions. Chiropractic addresses exclusively the vertebral subluxation.

ART. 189. CONTAGION AND INFECTION

Contagion and infection involve germs, viruses, bacteria, and other organisms, as penetrative information/F that are transmitted through direct or indirect contact from one host to another. If the natural genetic resistance of the body is lowered due to vertebral subluxations causing interference in the momentum of the transmission of innate impulses for coordination of activities, the body will have a decreased level of adaptability. This disturbance of momentum in transmission is due to a lack of ease (DIS-EASE) of the transmitting nerve cells and prevents all the parts of the body to be coherent and synchronized (Prin. 29, 30, 31a, 33). Since the innate law is limited due to the limitation of E/matter, it may be impossible to adapt the body without breaking a universal law (Prin. 24). Chiropractic is always about what is possible.

ART. 190. BLOOD POISON

Blood carries tissue cells (erythrocytes, leucocytes, phagocytes, etc.) and nutrients to the parts of the body for metabolism. Any of those cells floating in the blood have their own metabolism; their vitality may be unsound. This requires those cells to be adapted by the innate control for use in the body, if it is possible according to universal laws, to keep the content of the blood balanced. If there is a lack of adaptability from those cells, or if toxic substances are introduced into the blood, it could lead to blood poisoning. Since vertebral subluxations further increase the limitation of E/matter, it is imperative that chiropractors practice exclusively the chiropractic objective, which is to locate, analyze and facilitate the correction of vertebral subluxations for an innate-normal transmission of innate impulses.

ART. 191. IMMUNITY

Immunity involves the degree of adaptability of tissue cells, which is dependent upon innate-normal transmission of innate impulses for coordination of activities of body parts and upon the innate-normal radiation of innate rays/waves for sound metabolism. Immunity is directly proportional to the constructive survival value of the entire body *(See Art. 133, 134)*. It is manifested as an internal resistance to adverse information/F derived from invader organisms. Building immunity depends upon the innate-normal transmission of innate impulses and soundness of vitality of the tissue cells of the body. When all the parts of the body have coordinated activities (coherence) and are sound, the adaptability of the body is at its very best providing the internal resistance necessary to counteract the penetrative invasive information/F associated with poison. This means that when the body is without vertebral subluxations, manifesting its natural genetic resistance, and the environment of the tissue cells is adequate, it is less susceptible to poisons derived from epidemics, endemics or pandemics. It is important to understand the immense contribution that practicing the chiropractic objective adds to the transmission of innate impulses of the body (Prin. 31b, 32, 33), in order for the body to manifest its natural genetic resisitence.

Dr. Claude Lessard

REVIEW QUESTIONS FOR ARTICLES 182 - 191

1. Explain how air is an environmental factor.
2. Explain how climate is an environmental factor.
3. Explain how hygiene is an environmental factor.
4. What is effluvia and explain how it is an environmental factor.
5. Explain how germs are an environmental factor.
6. Are germs living organisms?
7. What law governs the component materials of germs?
8. What is a parasite?
9. How are parasites useful to the body of the host?
10. What are epidemics, endemics and pandemics?
11. Give the ADIO perspective of epidemics, endemics and pandemics.
12. Give the ADIO perspective of contagion and infection.
13. How can the body have blood poisoning?
14. How is immunity manifested in the body?

ART. 192. DIS-EASE AND ITS CAUSE IS CONTINUALLY IN A STATE OF FLUX

Articles 120 and 121, presented that the cause of DIS-EASE is always directly or indirectly due to vertebral subluxations. DIS-EASE is a condition of the transmitting E/matter (nerve cells) that does not have the property of ease. The tone of the nerve is too tense or too slack. This lack of ease (DIS-EASE) of the transmitting neurons interferes with the momentum of transmission of innate impulses and always leads to in-coordination of activities in the body (Prin. 30, 32). In chiropractic, it is always the direct or indirect result of vertebral subluxations (Prin. 31a). If there is no interference in transmission of innate impulses, there is a continuous adaptability from the body's E/matter and computation from the innate law (Prin. 33) to ensure coordination of actions of all the parts of the body in fulfilling their roles and purposes (Prin. 32). This occurs if it is possible according to universal laws (Prin. 24). This lack of ease (DIS-EASE) of the nerve tissues is caused by the vertebral subluxation and is located at site of the vertebral subluxation impinging the neurons, which interfere with the momentum in transmission of innate impulses. DIS-EASE leads to a lack of coordination of activities (incoherence) of body parts (Prin. 32). Confirming that interference with transmission of innate impulses causes incoordination of DIS-EASE (Prin. 30).

The innate law is about living things. Living organisms are maintained alive by the innate law. The human body is maintained alive by the innate law (Prin. 21). The human body is continually adapted, processed and reorganized by the innate law to be maintained alive moment by moment if it is possible according to universal laws (Prin. 23, 24). The body is always in a state of flux. For example, the body undergoes a turnover of cellular replacement at the rate of 330 billion cells every day.[35] These cells are replaced from all over the body, including bone, blood, muscles, skin, ligaments, vessels, organs, glands, etc. Therefore, a vertebral subluxation is also always in state of flux and it is never static. Remember that the body is vitalistic and not mechanistic. A vertebral subluxation is the loss of juxtaposition of two vertebrae that are living parts of the human body. The nerve that is affected is a living part of the human body. As such, those living tissues are continually adapted, processed and reorganized by the innate law (Prin. 23). When an adjustic thrust (which is a specific external educated information/F) is intentionally introduced into the body, it is with the understanding that the innate control may adapt this educated information/F into innate information/F to process a vertebral adjustment to correct a vertebral subluxation (Prin. 31b) if it is possible without breaking a universal law (Prin. 23, 24). The chiropractor's specific adjustic thrust is a fundamental of chiropractic's applied science through the application of principle 31a and 31b of chiropractic's basic science.

The continuous external invasive information/F are steadily interacting with the internal natural genetic resistance of the body to keep the body balanced. Since both are continuously occurring, they are also in a state of flux. Everything in the body is in a state of flux. For this reason, the recurrence of vertebral subluxation is also in a state a flux. The student may ask, "How do we prevent the recurrence of vertebral subluxations?" And the answer is, by locating, analyzing, and facilitating the correction of vertebral subluxations that are present at the moment of the chiropractic visit by the practice member in order to restore the transmission of innate impulses that will bring back the limitation of E/matter to its natural genetic level. When the vertebral subluxation is corrected, the momentum of transmission of innate impulses returns to innate-normal (Prin. 27), thereby satisfying the principle of coordination (Prin. 32). The internal resistance of the body is then strong enough to balance the concussion external information/F that could otherwise overcome the internal resistive information/F that would cause a vertebral subluxation.

---

35. Fischetti, M. & Christiansen, J. Our Bodies Replace Billions of Cells Every Day. "Scientific American". (April 1, 2021).

Dr. Claude Lessard

ART. 193. THE PHILOSOPHY OF ADAPTIVE BODY CHEMISTRY

This explanation pertains to the body's adaptability to invading toxins. It is given for the purpose of pointing to the 100%/perfect and complete innate software (Prin. 22, 33) that continually adapts, processes and reorganizes information/F and E/matter for use in the body, so that all parts of the body will have coordinated action (coherence) for mutual benefit (Prin. 23).

When toxins are present within the body, the innate control will process them accordingly through the organs and glands of the excretory systems only if it is possible according to universal laws (Prin. 24). Chiropractic does not address the effects of these processes. Chiropractic only addresses a specific cause of interference, which is the vertebral subluxation, to restore the momentum of the transmission of innate impulses used by the innate law to process the information/F and E/matter of the body. Chiropractic is only and always about cause. Chiropractic is never about effect (Prin. 31a, 31b, 32, 33). When a vertebral subluxation is corrected by the innate law (Prin. 31b), the momentum of the transmission of innate impulses is always restored, so that the instruction that is coded therein will be received in a timely manner by the body part receptor (Prin. 6). What happens after that is accomplished, are the manifestations of this restoration of momentum of the transmission of innate impulses. Sometimes it may be health enhancement and sometimes not. Sometimes is may be an increased performance and sometimes not. Sometimes it may be a better expression of human potential and sometimes not. Sometimes it may be getting well from sickness and sometimes not. Sometimes it may be an elimination of toxins that improves whatever may be going on in the body at the time, and sometimes not. These effects are specific physical manifestations of motion in living E/matter resulting from its expression of information/F (Prin. 13, 14, 15, 20, 21) that happens, sometimes.

Chiropractic is always about cause. Chiropractic is never concerned with effect. Let me repeat it again, chiropractic is without exception about cause. Chiropractic is never about effect. Chiropractic is always about cause.

ART. 194. ADAPTIVE BODY CHEMISTRY CYCLE AND PROCESSING OF TOXINS

Following the understanding of the previous article, the student is now directed to return to Article 129, including Fig. 20 and apply the complete in-coordination of activities cycle regardless of any and all manifestations of motion, which are deconstructive or reconstructive (Prin. 26) of living E/matter. The application of Fig. 20 becomes the blueprint that can be used for verifying whether or not the applied science of the principles continually keeps the practice of the chiropractic objective at cause. The regular use of this cycle will insure a thorough understanding of the preeminent importance to practice exclusively the chiropractic objective in order to remain at cause regardless of any of the circumstances of the chiropractic visit by the practice member.

ART. 195. IMBALANCE OF BODY CHEMISTRY

Interference in transmission momentum of innate impulses (Prin. 29) is always directly or indirectly due to vertebral subluxations (Prin. 31a). This interference will bring about in-coordination of activities of body parts (Prin. 30, 32). In-coordination of activities of body parts can manifests an imbalance of body chemistry. It is incumbent to apply the in-coordination of activities cycle to verify the predictions of the chiropractic objective in practice and its accurate innate computation. The student is strongly encouraged to practice exclusively the chiropractic objective, which is always at cause.

ART. 196. UN-ADAPTED BODY ACTIVITIES

Following the previous article, it is possible that the educated activities of a body part lack adaptability due to vertebral subluxations. The motion of un-adapted body parts will manifest in-coordination of activities (incoherence). This could possibly engender an imbalance of body chemistry that could poison the serous circulation of body chemistry *(See Art. 155)*. Once again it is incumbent to apply the in-coordination of activities cycle to verify the predictions of the chiropractic objective in practice and its accurate innate computation. The student is strongly encouraged to practice exclusively the chiropractic objective, which is always at cause.

ART. 197. STIMULATION

Stimulation comes from a stimulant that is an external information/F penetrating E/matter *(See Art. 117)*. This external penetrative information/F must be adapted, processed and computed by the innate law for use in the body within the limits of adaptation (Prin. 23, 24). If not, the innate control will act through the resistance of the body to prevent damage according to universal laws. If the external information/F overcomes the internal resistance of the body, it will cause a vertebral subluxation. The vertebral subluxation will then further increase the limitation of E/matter.

As a penetrative information/F, if the stimulant can be adapted and computed by the innate law, then the stimulation will be processed for use in the body (Prin. 23) or it will be resisted, which is an innate-normal function (Prin. 27). If the stimulation overcomes the internal resistance, it will cause a vertebral subluxation, which is an abnormal reaction (Prin. 31a).

Note that stimulation connotes an increase function different than innate-normal. It is never an innate function because the innate law is always normal and its function is always normal (Prin. 27). The innate law never stimulates since stimulation is always abnormal and requires adaptation within the limitation of E/matter (Prin. 24).

ART. 198. INHIBITION

Inhibition comes from inhibitors that is an external information/F penetrating E/matter. Inhibitors need to be adapted, processed and computed by the innate law in the same way as are stimulants. Stimulation and inhibition require adaptation since they are penetrative information/F *(See Art. 117)*. Inhibition follows the exact same process as stimulation. A body part that is adapted is neither stimulated nor inhibited, it is being reconstructed. A body part that is not adapted due to limitation of E/matter or vertebral subluxations, will express information/F accordingly and will be deconstructed due to the un-adapted penetrative universal information/F (Prin. 26). The student is once again reminded that it is important for the chiropractor to practice exclusively the chiropractic objective, which is always at cause.

ART. 199. APPLICATION OF THE CYCLES OF THE BODY'S ADAPTABILITY TO POISON

Here is an example of two flowcharts involved simultaneously, along with a multitude of other flowcharts. The first one demonstrates the normal innate adaptation in the form of ejection of the poison. The second demonstrates the normal innate adaptation in the form of repair from the poison's damage to the tissue cells through cellular replacement. These two flowcharts operate in conjunction with the innate-normal food cycle *(See Art. 126, Fig. 19)*.

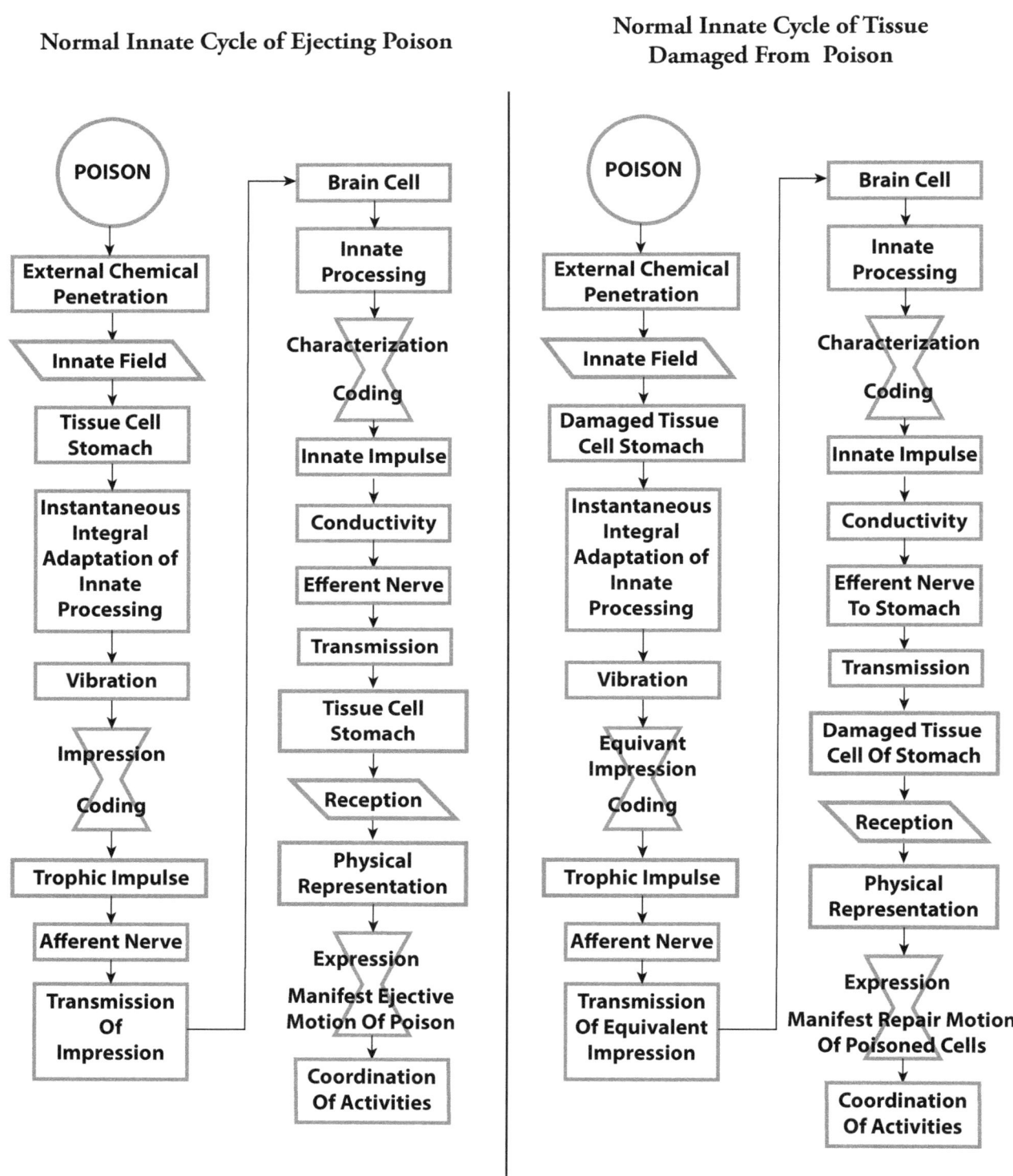

Fig. 29 Two examples of innate adaptation cycles of a stomach that has ingested poison.

These two cycles are examples of normal innate processing which highlight the adaptability of the body by the innate law according to universal laws (Prin. 24). Innate processing begins in the innate field as it adapts universal information/F (inforuns.) In both instances the body returns to its innate-normal cycles in a successful manner (Prin. 27). It also illustrates the amazing innate computation required under the innate control to adapt, process and govern the multitude of operational steps necessary for coordination of activities or every multi-billion cycles within the body simultaneously. This is what the chiropractors' participation is when they practice the chiropractic objective, which is to locate, analyze and facilitate the correction of vertebral subluxation for an innate-normal transmission of innate impulses. PERIOD.

ART. 200. APPLICATION OF CYCLES OF THE BODY'S UNADAPTABILITY TO POISON DUE TO LIMITATION OF E/MATTER

This complex cycle uses the abnormal complete cycle causing in-coordination of activities *(See Art. 124, Fig. 18)*. It is applied to illustrate the concussion of universal information/F that overcomes the internal natural genetic resistance of the body, which causes a vertebral subluxation that further increases the limitation of E/matter. This is the single most important flowchart for the student to memorize. This flowchart is applied to every concussion of information/F within the body. It is the basic genesis of locating, analyzing and facilitating the correction of vertebral subluxation.

The cycle of the body's un-adaptability to poison explains how the poison that is introduced in the body and is not excreted from the body will cause tissue damage and vertebral subluxation. It is an external invasive information/F overcoming the internal resistance of the body as a shock. This will further increase the limitation of E/matter thereby limiting the body's ability to compensate and adapt through cellular replacement. Repair of the body part will be impaired. Let the student note that the lack of ease (DIS-EASE) of the transmitting neuron will alter the momentum of the transmission of innate impulses, thus leading to in-coordination of activities of body parts (Prin. 29, 30, 31a, 32).

This cycle is compounded with the vertemere cycle showing a concussion of information/F where non-adapted external invasive infomation/F overcomes the internal innate natural genetic resistance of the body that causes a vertebral subluxation interfering with the momentum in transmission of innate impulses (Prin. 29, 30, 31a). The adaptability of the body is overcome due to the limitation of E/matter (Prin. 24) and the shock produced by the poison introduces an abnormal cycle of in-coordination of activities at the vertemere.

Within the flowchart of Fig. 20, the clear boxes represent the normal complete cycles for coordination of activities; the dark boxes represent a cycle from brain cell to the tissue cells of the vertemere, which is the region of the vertebra itself. It also demonstrates the unbalanced resistance resulting from a concussion of information/F (in this case the poison shock). This makes it a compound cycle for study. This is one of the most important cycles in the study of chiropractic, and the students should make themselves well acquainted with it. It is the only flowchart with immediate practical application as applied science, and it is the fundamental basis for the art of chiropractic analysis, which will be highlighted in Volume 4.

This flowchart explains the cause for the vertebral subluxation and why it does not get corrected in spite of the computation of information/F under the innate control. The interference with the momentum in transmission of innate impulses to the tissues of the vertemere increases the limitation of E/matter that prevents the process of a vertebral adjustment from the innate control that would be using the corrective vertebral muscles to move the articular facets of the vertebra within its normal juxtaposition. Fig. 20 demonstrates the in-coordination of the abnormal vertemere cycle due to the vertebral subluxation. This is the reason why the practice of the chiropractic objective today is the best way to prevent the vertebral subluxation of tomorrow. Chiropractic is always about what is possible.

Even though the innate processes are computing all information/F available, it cannot restore the vertebra to it proper juxtaposition due to the lack of momentum transmission of information/F to the vertemere. This means that the innate law is continually adapting information/F in order to process a vertebral adjustment within the limitations of E/matter.

When chiropractors analyze the state of the vertemere through ADIO analysis which employs muscle palpation to identify the myo-vectors of the working muscles that the innate law uses to process a vertebral adjustment (Prin. 31b), they introduce a specific adjustic thrust that could provide the added information/F necessary for the innate law to process a vertebral adjustment *(See Fig. 20)* to break out of the complete in-coordination of activities cycle. This is the basis for the ADIO analysis that I co-developed with Miguel Bolufer and its founder Reggie Gold, D.C., in the 1970s, in order to determine the location and analyze the myo-vectors of the subluxated vertebra. In volume 4, the reproduction of a few articles published in the late 1970s and early 1980s will be addressing the origin of this analysis. In Fig. 20, notice that the arrow going from the innate realm (field) directly to the tissue cell indicates the adaptation of the tissue cell for metabolism through innate rays/waves. Innate rays/waves are not addressed by chiropractic. Chiropractic only addresses interference in momentum of transmission of innate impulses from vertebral subluxations.

Abnormal Cycle of Body's Unadaptability to Poison Due to Limitation of E/Matter

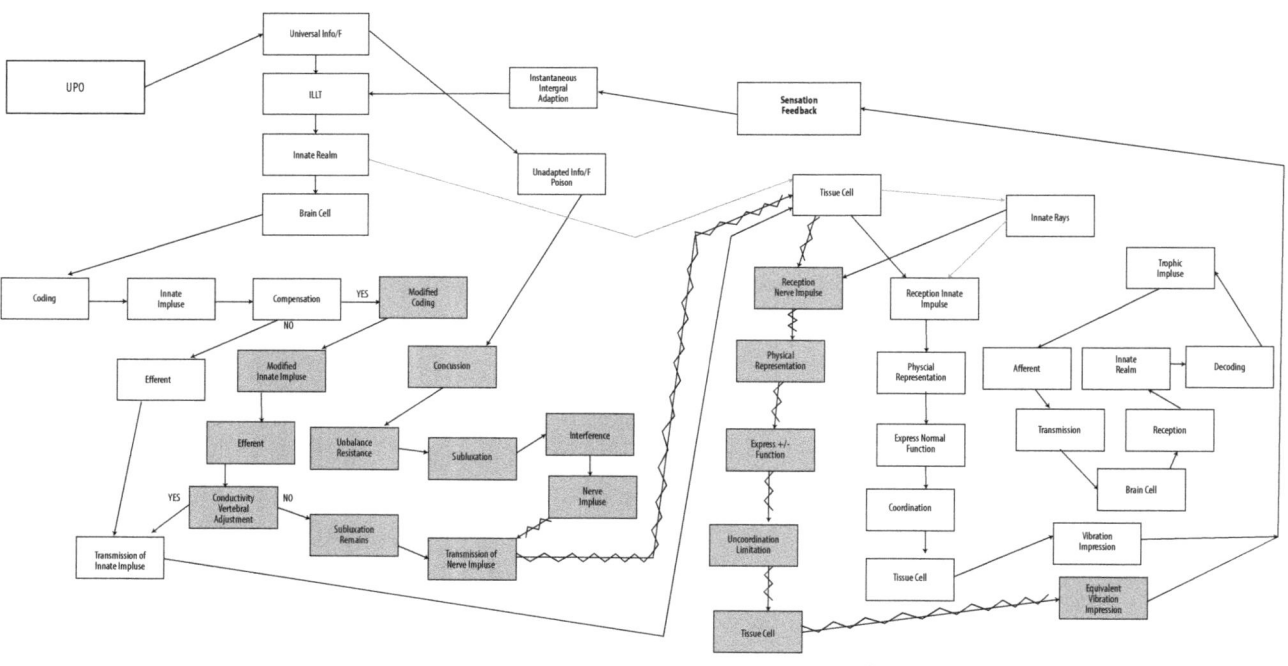

Fig. 30 is a flowchart showing poison as an external invasive information/F that may overcome the internal resistance of the body already caused by a vertebral subluxation that may cause a vertebral subluxation that interferes with the cycle of adaptability devolving into the abnormal cycle of un-adaptability to poison.

Note: Chiropractic asserts that the vertebral subluxation came first, directly or indirectly, causing a lack of ease (DIS-EASE) of the transmitting neurons (Prin. 30, 31a).

The cycle of the body's un-adaptability to poison due to limitation of E/matter demonstrates how a poison is an external penetrative information/F that can overcome the internal resistance of the body. This cycle is compounded with the vertemere cycle. Once again, the student is reminded that poison is here used as an example of a multitude of external invasive information/F that penetrate the body on a regular basis. Chiropractic does not address these penetrative information/F and how to prevent them. Chiropractic addresses exclusively the vertebral subluxation. Nothing more. Nothing less. Nothing else.

ART. 201. POISON IS ALWAYS AN EXTERNAL INVASIVE INFORMATION/F

Poison is an external invasive information/F that can overcome the internal resistance of the body. The ingestion of a poison by the body, which is an external invasive information/F, can cause a vertebral subluxation thereby further increasing the limitation of E/matter. External invasive information/F never limits the ability of the innate law to adapt, compute and process information/F. It is the limitation of E/matter that causes the body to be unable to adapt to the penetrative information/F (Prin. 24). The innate law is always 100%/perfect for any and all computation and processing. For example, if you give a triple shot of alcohol to a man who weighs 200 pounds, the innate law will adapt the external invasive shock to his body in order to eliminate the poison with minimum damage. However, if you give the same triple shot of alcohol to an infant, the external invasive shock may overcome the internal resistance of the infant's body and cause a vertebral subluxation to the extent that this action might be so overwhelming that the body of the infant may sustain maximum damage and could possibly die *(See Fig. 30)*.

Dr. Claude Lessard

REVIEW QUESTIONS FOR ARTICLES 192 - 201

1. Explain why DIS-EASE and its cause are always in a state of flux.
2. Explain the philosophy of adaptive body chemistry.
3. Which cycle is the blueprint of adaptive body chemistry?
4. Explain how can educated abilities of body parts lack adaptability?
5. Is stimulation an innate function?
6. What does inhibition require to not cause a vertebral subluxation?
7. Can a poison cause a vertebral subluxation?
8. Explain why and how poison can cause the body to die.

ART. 202. ADDICTION AND HABIT

The Merriam-Webster Dictionary defines *habit* as:

> **1:** A settled tendency or usual manner of behavior
>
> **2a:** An acquired mode of behavior that has become nearly or completely involuntary
>
> **2b:** ADDICTION a drug habit
>
> **2c:** A behavior pattern acquired by frequent repetition or physiologic exposure that shows itself in regularity or increased facility of performance

Human beings can only use their educated intelligence according to the development of their educated brain, over time (Prin. 6). Many people will repeat a certain act that is habit forming. It may be good or bad depending upon whether the habit is beneficial or not. To get your spine checked for vertebral subluxation regularly is a good habit as it is beneficial to the body as it has constructive survival values. To smoke a pack of cigarettes every day is a bad habit as it is detrimental to the body as it has deconstructive survival values. A habit can become "second" nature and the act is performed without thinking about it. However, the beginning of forming a habit always involves the educated intelligence of the individual, which is the capability of the educated brain to function. It is either a function of the educated brain or it is a function of the innate law, which in this case, would violate principle 25. This is impossible. Chiropractic is always about what is possible. Therefore, one who makes a bad choice can initiate the beginning of forming a bad habit. Human beings must, ultimately, take responsibility for their choice making through conscious discernment from an ADIO or OIBU worldview.

As such, a habit good or bad is an OIBU act from an individual using the portion of the educated brain that we call the will. Once a habit is formed, it may develop into an a good or bad addiction. This is because the innate law will adapt the body by processing the body chemistry necessary to counteract the substance that is involved in the addiction in order to neutralize it. If the habit of using substances continues, over time the body will crave the substance due to the chemical antidote that creates an imbalance in the body chemistry. The innate law is always a normal 100%/perfect software and will adapt, compute and process all the body chemistry necessary moment by moment, regardless of the substances involved according to universal laws (Prin. 22, 23, 24, 27). The imbalance of body chemistry is always due to limitation of E/matter, and that includes the limitation of the physical educated brain. For that reason, it requires great effort of the will from the educated brain to break a habit and may call for a great amount of time, especially for addiction.

If vertebral subluxations are present in the body further compromising the limitation of E/matter, it will be much more difficult to change a habit. From an ADIO perspective in Article 200, it is demonstrated how a poison can only be eliminated if a vertebral adjustment is processed by the innate law to correct a vertebral subluxation in order to restore the momentum in transmission of innate impulses (Prin. 31a, 31b). It underscores the importance for chiropractors to exclusively practice the chiropractic objective, which is always at cause.

ART. 204. MEDICATION HABITS AND PAIN KILLERS ADDICTION

Every medication has effects upon the body, not side effects. Side effects are what our educated intelligence does not want the drug to do. However, our educated intelligence does not know the effects a drug will have on any particular body, because everyone is different and unique.

Drugs, whether illicit or legally prescribed, belong to the OIBU approach to life. The OIBU worldview is when the educated intelligence, through its own egoistic addiction, assumes the governance of the myriad body chemistry processes, which is the normal function of the 100%/perfect innate law The usage of drugs interferes with natural body chemistry and acts as poisons to the body by either stimulating or inhibiting its physiological functions. They have far reaching effects, way beyond the immediate educated desired one. Prolonged usage of those drugs will form habits and possible addictions that will carry deconstructive survival values in the long run, further compromising to the limitation of E/matter. Chiropractic does not address this type of OIBU interference with physiological functions. Chiropractic addresses exclusively the vertebral subluxation.

ART. 205. 100%/PERFECT INSTANTANEOUS INTEGRAL ADAPTATION

Instantaneous integral adaptation is 100%/perfect innate computing process of every universal computation moment by moment in living organisms according to universal laws (Prin. 22, 23, 24). This innate process takes place within the 100%/perfect innate realm; it is strictly non-material; it is a vitalistic process; it is a non-discrete process occurring in the innate field in order to adapt the interoperability of an organism for use in its body and maintain it alive if it is possible according to universal laws (Prin. 21, 23, 24). It is the universal cycle of change that requires reconstruction from the innate law governing adaptation to maintain the structural molecular integrity of living E/matter (Prin. 26). It is part of the universal cycle of change intrinsic within the normal complete cycle *(See Vol. 1, Fig. 5, 6, 7)*. When organic living E/matter has reached its complete limitation of adaptability, it is no longer alive and the deconstruction aspect of the universal cycle of change takes over. The universal principle of organization deconstructs and breaks down the molecular structure E/matter to its most stable state, which is the atom.

The innate-normal function (Prin. 27) of this instantaneous integral process as a 100%/perfect software (Prin. 33) is always 100%/perfect. Its innate program is continually propagated through the ongoing generation of each species intrinsic within the genetic code of living E/matter with survival values, which is a fundamental principle in the evolutionary aspect of E/matter. 100%/perfect instantaneous integral adaptation consists of an unlimited innate software process adapting, computing and coding information/F within E/matter moment by moment, in contrast to the limited hardware used to process the information/F of living E/matter. We observe instantaneous integral adaptation processing of information/F by the expression of E/matter and its manifestation (Prin. 13, 14), which is called adaptation. It is due to the adaptability of E/matter by the innate law.

The innate law is a 100%/perfect and normal software (Prin. 22, 27, 33). Since it is perfect and complete, it is unlimited and it never changes. It always instantaneously and flawlessly adapts, computes, and codes the information/F involved and E/matter within the circumstantial reconstructive process according to the adaptability of the living organism moment by moment (Prin. 23, 24).

However, the universal cycle of change is unceasingly going on within E/matter. The universal information/F is consistently furnished through the principle of continuous supply and computation to all E/matter by the universal principle of organization (Prin. 33), thus deconstructing its structural form causing it to break down toward its most stable state, the atom (Prin. 26). For this reason, adaptation is necessary in order to maintain the E/matter of organism alive, if it is possible, according to universal laws (Prin. 21, 23, 24). It is precisely here that we notice the distinction between non-living and living E/matter. For example, if a fence builder uses a sledgehammer to drive posts into the soil, overtime the handle of the sledge hammer will wear down; yet the hands of the fence builder will grow a callous as an adaptive process by the innate law to protect the hands. This is as opposed to the wear and tear exerted on the wooden handle of the sledgehammer (Prin. 26). This amazing process of reconstruction of living E/matter is due to the instantaneous integral adaptation from the 100%/perfect and complete software, called the innate law of living things, which is immediately computing and coding information/F and E/matter that reconstructs the hands by growing a callous for body use (Prin. 23). And when living E/matter has reached its limits of adaptability, it is then deconstructed by the universal information/F that are no longer adapted by the innate control according to universal laws (Prin. 24).

The student is reminded of the importance to practice the chiropractic objective exclusively in order to restore the momentum in transmission innate impulses (Prin. 31 b) because even though the 100%/perfect instantaneous integral adaptation of the innate law software occurs immediately, the innate control is limited by the limitations of E/matter hardware (Prin. 24), which the vertebral subluxation further compromise. Philosophically, it has some far-reaching implications that literally and possibly mean that the unfolding of the species for future generations will inherit constructive survival values for a continuous higher level of adaptability since the innate control always adapts information/F and E/matter for the body only if it is possible according to universal laws.

ART. 206. ADAPTATION

Adaptation is the physical process that takes place as the manifestation of 100%/perfect instantaneous integral adaptation, as the expression of innate rays/waves for cell metabolism (cellular soundness of vitality), and innate impulses for coordination of activities of body parts (Prin. 23) according to universal laws (Prin. 24). It is the physical representation of it. It is a continuous process unceasingly varying. It is never constant. It is always changing. Adaptation is an innate function, which is normal (Prin. 27) with universal values for all living cells within the limitations of E/matter (Prin. 1, 20, 24).

Adaptation happens either quickly or overtime depending of the state of living E/matter (Prin. 6). For example, when a person is exposed to a virus, certain changes occur to empower the body to resist the invasive information/F and protect it from harm. It may include a variety of changes in body temperature, in body chemistry within the blood, in fluidity of serous circulation, in vascular permeability, etc. The body develops immunity, which possesses constructive survival values, through those changes. It becomes part and parcel of the evolutionary process of the species for posterity. Adaptation is the universal principle of change always according to universal laws. It is a physical process that takes place within a species and causes it to evolve according to its genetic code and its living circumstances. It is a physical manifestation of E/matter of 100%/perfect instantaneous integral adaptation, from the innate control, if it is possible according to universal laws (Prin. 5, 22, 24).

The living body is truly a universal computer equipped with a 100%/perfect, complete, and always current innate-software that continually adapts and processes information/F and E/matter for use in the body-hardware so that all parts of the body will have coordinated action for mutual benefit (Prin. 23, 32, 33).

ART. 207. GENETIC SUSCEPTIBILITY

Genetic susceptibility is a particular sensitivity to a specific agent that is inherited from genetic variations of a parent. It is part of the limitations of E/matter of the offspring that may or may not contribute to weakening body resistance regarding the specific agent. It is dependent on multiple factors, like vertebral subluxations, genetic modifiers, environment, circumstances, lifestyle, etc. The innate law will always adapt the body of a living thing according to universal laws, which includes the law of genetics (Prin. 24). Chiropractic recognizes the "sometimes" susceptibility of the living body. From an ADIO viewpoint, it is the individual's responsibility to make elegant educated choices regarding the factors involved in body resistance. Chiropractic does not address those factors. For the student, it once again underscores the importance to practice exclusively the chiropractic objective, which is, the location, the analysis and the facilitation of the correction of vertebral subluxations for an innate-normal transmission of innate impulses.

REVIEW QUESTIONS FOR ARTICLES 202 - 207

1. Explain addiction and habit.
2. What is the distinction between medication and poison?
3. Explain pain killer addiction.
4. Explain instantaneous integral adaptation.
5. Explain adaptation as related to survival value and evolution.
6. What is the value produced by adaptation which is transmitted to posterity?
7. What kind of adaptation is inherited by posterity?
8. What are some of the factors involved that may weaken body resistance?
9. Adaptation is the universal principle of what?
10. Explain genetic susceptibility.
11. Who is responsible to make elegant educated choices regarding lifestyle?

This concludes Volume Two.

Proceed to Volume Three.

BIBLIOGRAPHY VOL 2:

1. Strauss, Joseph. "The Green Book Commentaries, Vol. XIV (1927) Chiropractic Text Book." Levittown, PA: Foundation for Advancement of Chiropractic Education. (2002) p. 17

2. Palmer, B.J., "The Science of Chiropractic, Its Principles and Philosophies." 4th ed., Davenport, IA: The Palmer School of Chiropractic-Chiropractic Fountain Head. (1920) p. 12

25. Palmer, D.D., "Text-Book of the Science, Art, and Philosophy of Chiropractic for Students and Practioners." Portland, OR: Portland Printing House Company. (1910) p.7

26. Selye, H. "The Stress of LIfe." New York: McGraw-Hill Book Company, Inc. (1956) p.1

27. Zygomatic Nerve. https://anatomy.co.uk/zygomatic-nerve/ (1999-2003) June 2024

28. "Impulse and Momentum." The Physics Hypertextbook. physics.info/momentum/summary.shtml (1998-2024) June 2024

29. "Momentum." wordnetweb.princeton.edu June 2024

30. Palmer, Mabel H., "Anatomy." 4th ed., Davenport, IA: The Palmer School of Chiropractic- Chiropractic Fountain Head. (1920) p.317

31. Lessard, Claude. "Timed Out: Chiropractic." Self-published, Claude Lessard D.C. (2002) p. 39

32. Palmer, B.J. "My Message Analyzed."

33. "Earth" science.nasa.gov/earth/facts June 2024

34. Buckingham, L.J., & Ashby, B. (2022) Coevolutionary Theory of hosts and parasites. "Journal of Evolutionary Biology." 35, 205-224. DOI: 10.1111/jeb.13981

35. Fischetti, M. & Christiansen, J. Our Bodies Replace Billions of Cells Every Day. "Scientific American." (April 1, 2021) https://www.scientificamerican.com/article/our-bodies-replace-billions-of-cells-every-day/ June 2024

The 2027 Chiropractic Textbook Volume 2

CURRICULUM VITAE
DR. CLAUDE LESSARD

- B.S. Limestone College, Gaffney, S.C. 1977
- Doctor Of Chiropractic Degree, Sherman College Of Straight Chiropractic (S.C.S.C), Spartanburg, S.C. 1977
- Internship, S.C.S.C. 1977
- Recipient Of The B.J. Palmer Chiropractic Philosophy Distinction Award, S.C.S.C. 1977
- Diplomate Of The National Board Of Chiropractic Examiners
- Certified For Preliminary Professional Education #C35301, Commonwealth Of Pennsylvania
- Commonwealth Of Pennsylvania License #DC-1702-L
- Co-Founder And Charter Member Of ADIO Institute Of Straight Chiropractic 1978
- Student Referral Counselor, ADIO I.S.C. 1978-1981
- Assistant Professor Of Chiropractic Philosophy, ADIO I.S.C. 1978-1980
- Co-Developer of The ADIO Analysis 1978
- Administrative Dean Of ADIO I.S.C. 1979-1980
- Associate Professor Of Chiropractic Technique, ADIO I.S.C. 1980-1981
- Director Community Health Center, ADIO I.S.C. 1980-1981
- Member Chiropractic Life Fellowship Of Pennsylvania
- Member Of The Federation Of Straight Chiropractors Organization (F.S.C.O.)
- Graduate Of Church Ministry Program, St. Charles Borromeo Seminary 1983-1987
- Certified Myotech Examiner
- Chiropractor Of The Month Award, Markson Management Services, 1988
- Chiropractor Of The Year Award, Markson Management Services, 1992
- Post Graduate Course Of Study In Applied Spinal Biomechanics From The Aragona Spinal Biomechanic Engineering Laboratory, Inc. 1992
- Chiropractor Of The Year Award, Quest Management Systems, 1993
- Member Of The Distinguished Board Of Regents, S.C.S.C. Since 1993
- Member Of Parker Chiropractic Resources Foundation
- Chair And Co-Author Of "Spirit Of '76", S.C.S.C. 1996
- Founder Of Clients Association For Chiropractic Education (C.A.C.E.), 1997
- Licensed Private Pilot, Single Engine Airplanes Land, 1998
- Founder Of Lessard Institute For Chiropractic Clients, 1998
- Recipient Of The Spirit Of Sherman College Of Straight Chiropractic Award, 1999
- Licensed Pilot, Instrument Airplanes, 2000
- Author Of "Chiropractic.... Amazing Isn't It?" 2003
- Chiropractor Of The Year, S.C.S.C., 2006
- Motion De Felicitations, Ville De Ste. Anne De Beaupre, Resolutions 5553-09-06., 2006
- Pulstar Examiner, 2008

- Translation Of "Chiropractic…Amazing Isn't It?" In French, 2008
- Translation Of "Chiropractic…Amazing Isn't It?" In Spanish, 2009
- Autor Del Libro "Quiropraxia No Es Asombrosa?" 2010
- Auteur Du Livre "La Chiropratique, Incroyable N'est-Ce Pas?" 2012
- Author Of Blue Book "A New Look At Chiropractic Basic Science" 2017
- Autor Del Libro Azul "Una Mirada A La Scienca Basica Quiropractica" 2019
- Keynote Speaker At Sherman College Of Chiropractic International Research And Philosophy Symposium, 2019
- Author Of "Chiropractic, Amazing Isn't It- Workbook" 2020
- Author of Blue Book "Timed Out: Chiropractic" 2022
- Autor Del Libro Azul "Quiropráctica Reseteada" 2023
- Author Of "The 2027 Chiropractic Textbook Volume 1" 2024
- Autor Del Libro "Libro deTexto de Quiropráctica 2027 Volume 1" 2024

Dr. Claude Lessard

www.ingramcontent.com/pod-product-compliance
Lightning Source LLC
LaVergne TN
LVHW070603070526
838199LV00011B/471